PALEO DIET RECIPES 2021

TASTY RECIPES EASY TO MAKE FOR BEGINNERS

CECILIA BRIDGEWATER

Table of Contents

Grilled Strip Steaks with Grated Root Vegetable Hash 7
Asian Beef and Vegetable Stir-Fry 9
Cedar-Planked Filets with Asian Slather and Slaw 11
Pan-Seared Tri-Tip Steaks with Cauliflower Peperonata 14
Flat-Iron Steaks au Poivre with Mushroom-Dijon Sauce 16
Steaks 16
Sauce 16
Grilled Flat-Iron Steaks with Chipotle-Caramelized Onions and Salsa Salad 19
Steaks 19
Salsa Salad 19
Caramelized Onions 19
Grilled Ribeyes with Herbed Onion and Garlic "Butter" 22
Ribeye Salad with Grilled Beets 24
Korean-Style Short Ribs with Sautéed Ginger Cabbage 26
Beef Short Ribs with Citrus-Fennel Gremolata 29
Ribs 29
Pan-Roasted Squash 29
Gremolata 29
Swedish-Style Beef Patties with Mustard-Dill Cucumber Salad 32
Cucumber Salad 32
Beef Patties 32
Smothered Beefburgers on Arugula with Roasted Root Vegetables 36
Grilled Beefburgers with Sesame-Crusted Tomatoes 39
Burgers on a Stick with Baba Ghanoush Dipping Sauce 41
Smoky Stuffed Sweet Peppers 43
Bison Burgers with Cabernet Onions and Arugula 45
Bison and Lamb Meat Loaf on Chard and Sweet Potatoes 48
Apple-Currant-Sauced Bison Meatballs with Zucchini Pappardelle 51
Meatballs 51
Apple-Currant Sauce 51
Zucchini Pappardelle 51

Bison-Porcini Bolognese with Roasted Garlic Spaghetti Squash..................54
Bison Chili con Carne..................56
Moroccan-Spiced Bison Steaks with Grilled Lemons..................58
Herbes de Provence-Rubbed Bison Sirloin Roast..................59
Coffee-Braised Bison Short Ribs with Tangerine Gremolata and Celery Root Mash 61
Marinade..................61
Braise..................61
Beef Bone Broth..................64
Tunisian Spice-Rubbed Pork Shoulder with Spicy Sweet Potato Fries..................66
Pork 66
Fries 66
Cuban Grilled Pork Shoulder..................68
Italian Spice-Rubbed Pork Roast with Vegetables..................71
Slow Cooker Pork Mole..................73
Caraway-Spiced Pork and Squash Stew..................75
Fruit-Stuffed Top Loin Roast with Brandy Sauce..................77
Roast..................77
Brandy Sauce..................77
Porchetta-Style Pork Roast..................80
Tomatillo-Braised Pork Loin..................82
Apricot-Stuffed Pork Tenderloin..................84
Herb-Crusted Pork Tenderloin with Crispy Garlic Oil..................86
Indian-Spiced Pork with Coconut Pan Sauce..................87
Pork Scaloppini with Spiced Apples and Chestnuts..................88
Pork Fajita Stir-Fry..................91
Pork Tenderloin with Port and Prunes..................92
Moo Shu-Style Pork in Lettuce Cups with Quick Pickled Vegetables..................94
Pickled Vegetables..................94
Pork 94
Pork Chops with Macadamias, Sage, Figs, and Mashed Sweet Potatoes..................96
Skillet-Roasted Rosemary-Lavender Pork Chops with Grapes and Toasted Walnuts
..................98
Pork Chops alla Fiorentina with Grilled Broccoli Rabe..................100
Escarole-Stuffed Pork Chops..................102
Pork Chops with a Dijon-Pecan Crust..................105

Walnut-Crusted Pork with Blackberry Spinach Salad 106
Pork Schnitzel with Sweet-and-Sour Red Cabbage 108
Cabbage.. 108
Pork 108

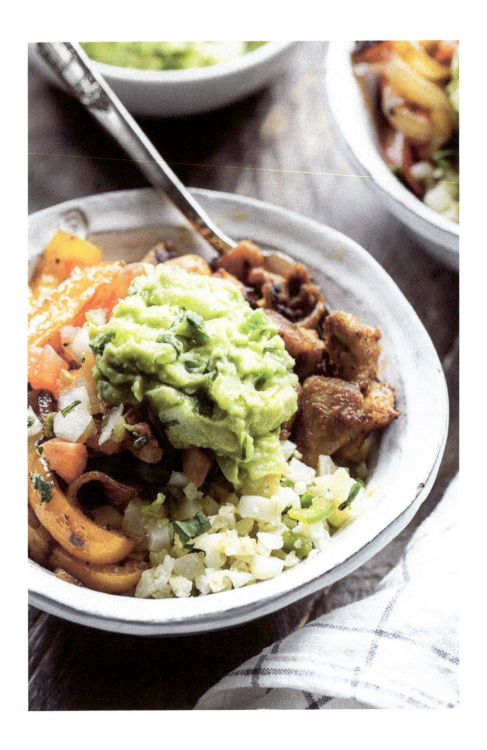

GRILLED STRIP STEAKS WITH GRATED ROOT VEGETABLE HASH

PREP: 20 minutes STAND: 20 minutes GRILL: 10 minutes STAND: 5 minutes MAKES: 4 servings

STRIP STEAKS HAVE A VERY TENDER TEXTURE, AND THE SMALL STRIP OF FAT ON ONE SIDE OF THE STEAK GETS CRISP AND SMOKY ON THE GRILL. MY THINKING ABOUT ANIMAL FAT HAS CHANGED SINCE MY FIRST BOOK. IF YOU ARE FAITHFUL TO THE BASIC PRINCIPLES OF THE PALEO DIET® AND KEEP SATURATED FATS WITHIN 10 TO 15 PERCENT OF YOUR DAILY CALORIES, IT WILL NOT INCREASE YOUR RISK OF HEART DISEASE—AND IN FACT, THE OPPOSITE MAY BE TRUE. NEW INFORMATION SUGGESTS THAT ELEVATIONS IN LDL CHOLESTEROL MAY ACTUALLY REDUCE SYSTEMIC INFLAMMATION, WHICH IS A RISK FACTOR FOR HEART DISEASE.

- 3 tablespoons extra virgin olive oil
- 2 tablespoons grated fresh horseradish
- 1 teaspoon finely shredded orange peel
- ½ teaspoon ground cumin
- ½ teaspoon black pepper
- 4 strip steaks (also called top loin), cut about 1 inch thick
- 2 medium parsnips, peeled
- 1 large sweet potato, peeled
- 1 medium turnip, peeled
- 1 or 2 shallots, finely chopped
- 2 cloves garlic, minced
- 1 tablespoon snipped fresh thyme

1. In a small bowl stir together 1 tablespoon of the oil, horseradish, orange peel, cumin, and ¼ teaspoon of the

pepper. Spread the mixture over steaks; cover and let stand at room temperature for 15 minutes.

2. Meanwhile for hash, using a box grater or a food processor fitted with the shredding blade, shred the parsnips, sweet potato, and turnip. Place shredded vegetables in a large bowl; add shallot(s). In a small bowl combine the remaining 2 tablespoons oil, the remaining ¼ teaspoon pepper, garlic, and thyme. Drizzle over vegetables; toss to mix thoroughly. Fold a 36×18-inch piece of heavy foil in half to make a double thickness of foil that measures 18×18 inches. Place vegetable mixture in the center of the foil; bring up opposite edges of foil and seal with a double fold. Fold remaining edges to completely enclose the vegetables, leaving space for steam to build.

3. For a charcoal or gas grill, place steaks and foil packet on the grill rack directly over medium heat. Cover and grill steaks for 10 to 12 minutes for medium rare (145°F) or 12 to 15 minutes for medium (160°F), turning once halfway through grilling. Grill packet for 10 to 15 minutes or until vegetables are tender. Let steaks stand for 5 minutes while vegetables finish cooking. Divide vegetable hash among four serving plates; top with steaks.

ASIAN BEEF AND VEGETABLE STIR-FRY

PREP: 30 minutes COOK: 15 minutes MAKES: 4 servings

FIVE-SPICE POWDER IS A SALT-FREE SPICE BLEND USED WIDELY IN CHINESE COOKING. IT CONSISTS OF EQUAL PARTS GROUND CINNAMON, CLOVES, FENNEL SEEDS, STAR ANISE, AND SZECHWAN PEPPERCORNS.

- 1½ pounds boneless beef top sirloin steak or boneless beef round steak, cut 1 inch thick
- 1½ teaspoons five-spice powder
- 3 tablespoons refined coconut oil
- 1 small red onion, cut into thin wedges
- 1 small bunch asparagus (about 12 ounces), trimmed and cut into 3-inch pieces
- 1½ cups julienne-cut orange and/or yellow carrots
- 4 cloves garlic, minced
- 1 teaspoon finely shredded orange peel
- ¼ cup fresh orange juice
- ¼ cup Beef Bone Broth (see recipe) or no-salt-added beef broth
- ¼ cup white wine vinegar
- ¼ to ½ teaspoon crushed red pepper
- 8 cups coarsely shredded napa cabbage
- ½ cup unsalted slivered almonds or unsalted coarsely chopped cashews, toasted (see tip, page 57)

1. If desired, partially freeze beef for easier slicing (about 20 minutes). Cut beef into very thin slices. In a large bowl toss together beef and five-spice powder. In a large wok or extra-large skillet heat 1 tablespoon of the coconut oil over medium-high heat. Add half the beef; cook and stir for 3 to 5 minutes or until browned. Transfer beef to a bowl. Repeat with the remaining beef and another 1

tablespoon oil. Transfer beef to the bowl with the other cooked beef.

2. In the same wok add the remaining 1 tablespoon oil. Add onion; cook and stir for 3 minutes. Add asparagus and carrots; cook and stir for 2 to 3 minutes or until vegetables are crisp-tender. Add garlic; cook and stir for 1 minute more.

3. For sauce, in a small bowl combine orange peel, orange juice, Beef Bone Broth, vinegar, and crushed red pepper. Add sauce and all the beef with juices in bowl to vegetables in wok. Cook and stir for 1 to 2 minutes or until heated through. Using a slotted spoon, transfer beef vegetables to a large bowl. Cover to keep warm.

4. Cook the sauce, uncovered, over medium heat for 2 minutes. Add cabbage; cook and stir for 1 to 2 minutes or until cabbage is just wilted. Divide cabbage and any cooking juices among four serving plates. Top evenly with beef mixture. Sprinkle with nuts.

CEDAR-PLANKED FILETS WITH ASIAN SLATHER AND SLAW

SOAK: 1 hour PREP: 40 minutes GRILL: 13 minutes STAND: 10 minutes MAKES: 4 servings.

NAPA CABBAGE IS SOMETIMES CALLED CHINESE CABBAGE. IT HAS BEAUTIFUL, CRINKLY CREAM-COLOR LEAVES WITH BRIGHT YELLOW-GREEN TIPS. IT HAS A DELICATE, MILD FLAVOR AND TEXTURE—QUITE DIFFERENT THAN THE WAXY LEAVES OF ROUND-HEADED CABBAGE—AND NOT SURPRISINGLY, IS A NATURAL IN ASIAN-STYLE DISHES.

1 large cedar plank
¼ ounce dried shiitake mushrooms
¼ cup walnut oil
2 teaspoons minced fresh ginger
2 teaspoons crushed red pepper
1 teaspoon crushed Szechwan peppercorns
¼ teaspoon five-spice powder
4 cloves garlic, minced
4 4- to 5-ounce beef tenderloin steaks, cut ¾ to 1 inch thick
Asian Slaw (see recipe, below)

1. Place grill plank in water; weight down and soak for at least 1 hour.

2. Meanwhile, for Asian slather, in a small bowl pour boiling water over dried shiitake mushrooms; let stand for 20 minutes to rehydrate. Drain mushrooms and place in a food processor. Add walnut oil, ginger, crushed red pepper, Szechuan peppercorns, five-spice powder, and garlic. Cover and process until mushrooms are minced and ingredients are combined; set aside.

3. Drain grill plank. For a charcoal grill, arrange medium-hot coals around perimeter of grill. Place plank on grill rack directly over coals. Cover and grill for 3 to 5 minutes or until plank begins to crackle and smoke. Place steaks on grill rack directly over coals; grill for 3 to 4 minutes or until seared. Transfer steaks to the plank, seared sides up. Place plank in center of grill. Divide Asian Slather among steaks. Cover and grill for 10 to 12 minutes or until an instant-read thermometer inserted horizontally into the steaks reads 130°F. (For a gas grill, preheat grill. Reduce heat to medium. Place drained plank on grill rack; cover and grill for 3 to 5 minutes or until plank begins to crackle and smoke. Place steaks on grill rack for 3 to 4 minutes or until seared. Transfer steaks to the plank, seared sides up. Adjust grill for indirect cooking; place plank with steaks over the burner that is turned off. Divide slather among steaks. Cover and grill for 10 to 12 minutes or until an instant-read thermometer inserted horizontally into the steaks reads 130°F.)

4. Remove steaks from the grill. Cover steaks loosely with foil; let stand for 10 minutes. Cut steaks into ¼-inch-thick slices. Serve steak over Asian Slaw.

Asian Slaw: In a large bowl combine 1 medium head napa cabbage, thinly sliced; 1 cup finely shredded red cabbage; 2 carrots, peeled and cut into julienne strips; 1 red or yellow sweet pepper, seeded and very thinly sliced; 4 scallions, thinly bias-sliced; 1 to 2 serrano chiles, seeded and minced (see tip); 2 tablespoons chopped cilantro; and 2 tablespoons chopped mint. For dressing, in a food processor or blender combine 3 tablespoons fresh lime juice, 1 tablespoon grated fresh ginger, 1 cloves minced garlic, and ⅛ teaspoon five-spice powder. Cover and process until smooth. With the processor running, gradually add ½ cup walnut oil and process until smooth. Add 1 scallion, thinly bias-sliced, to the dressing. Drizzle over slaw and toss to coat.

PAN-SEARED TRI-TIP STEAKS WITH CAULIFLOWER PEPERONATA

PREP: 25 minutes COOK: 25 minutes MAKES: 2 servings

PEPERONATA IS TRADITIONALLY A SLOW-ROASTED RAGU OF SWEET PEPPERS WITH ONION, GARLIC, AND HERBS. THIS QUICK SAUTÉED VERSION—MADE HEARTIER WITH CAULIFLOWER—ACTS AS BOTH RELISH AND SIDE DISH.

- 2 4- to 6-ounce tri-tip steaks, cut ¾ to 1 inch thick
- ¾ teaspoon black pepper
- 2 tablespoons extra virgin olive oil
- 2 red and/or yellow sweet peppers, seeded and sliced
- 1 shallot, thinly sliced
- 1 teaspoon Mediterranean Seasoning (see recipe)
- 2 cups small cauliflower florets
- 2 tablespoons balsamic vinegar
- 2 teaspoons snipped fresh thyme

1. Pat steaks dry with paper towels. Sprinkle steaks with ¼ teaspoon of the black pepper. In a large skillet heat 1 tablespoon of the oil over medium-high heat. Add steaks to skillet; reduce heat to medium. Cook steaks for 6 to 9 minutes for medium rare (145°F), turning occasionally. (If meat browns too quickly, reduce heat.) Remove steaks from skillet; cover loosely with foil to keep warm.

2. For the peperonata, add the remaining 1 tablespoon oil to the skillet. Add the sweet peppers and shallot. Sprinkle with Mediterranean Seasoning. Cook over medium heat about 5 minutes or until peppers are softened, stirring occasionally. Add cauliflower, balsamic vinegar, thyme,

and the remaining ½ teaspoon black pepper. Cover and cook for 10 to 15 minutes or until cauliflower is tender, stirring occasionally. Return steaks to skillet. Spoon peperonata mixture over steaks. Serve immediately.

FLAT-IRON STEAKS AU POIVRE WITH MUSHROOM-DIJON SAUCE

PREP: 15 minutes COOK: 20 minutes MAKES: 4 servings

THIS FRENCH-INSPIRED STEAK WITH MUSHROOM SAUCE CAN BE ON THE TABLE IN JUST OVER 30 MINUTES—WHICH MAKES IT A GREAT CHOICE FOR A QUICK WEEKNIGHT MEAL.

STEAKS
- 3 tablespoons extra virgin olive oil
- 1 pound small asparagus spears, trimmed
- 4 6-ounce flat-iron (boneless beef shoulder top blade) steaks*
- 2 tablespoons snipped fresh rosemary
- 1½ teaspoons cracked black pepper

SAUCE
- 8 ounces sliced fresh mushrooms
- 2 cloves garlic, minced
- ½ cup Beef Bone Broth (see recipe)
- ¼ cup dry white wine
- 1 tablespoon Dijon-Style Mustard (see recipe)

1. In a large skillet heat 1 tablespoon of the oil over medium-high heat. Add asparagus; cook for 8 to 10 minutes or until crisp-tender, turning spears occasionally so they don't burn. Transfer asparagus to a plate; cover with foil to keep warm.

2. Sprinkle steaks with rosemary and pepper; rub in with your fingers. In the same skillet heat the remaining 2 tablespoons oil over medium-high heat. Add steaks; reduce heat to medium. Cook for 8 to 12 minutes for medium rare (145°F), turning meat occasionally. (If meat

browns too quickly, reduce heat.) Remove meat from skillet, reserving drippings. Cover steaks loosely with foil to keep warm.

3. For sauce, add mushrooms and garlic to drippings in skillet; cook until tender, stirring occasionally. Add broth, wine, and Dijon-Style Mustard. Cook over medium heat, scraping up the browned bits in bottom of skillet. Bring to boiling; cook for 1 minute more.

4. Divide the asparagus among four dinner plates. Top with steaks; spoon sauce over the steaks.

*Note: If you can't find 6-ounce flat-iron steaks, purchase two 8- to 12-ounce steaks and cut them in half to make four steaks.

GRILLED FLAT-IRON STEAKS WITH CHIPOTLE-CARAMELIZED ONIONS AND SALSA SALAD

PREP: 30 minutes MARINATE: 2 hours BAKE: 20 minutes COOL: 20 minutes GRILL: 45 minutes MAKES: 4 servings

FLAT-IRON STEAK IS A RELATIVELY NEW CUT DEVELOPED JUST A FEW YEARS AGO. CUT FROM THE FLAVORFUL CHUCK SECTION NEAR THE SHOULDER BLADE, IT IS SURPRISINGLY TENDER AND TASTES MUCH MORE EXPENSIVE THAN IT IS—WHICH LIKELY ACCOUNTS FOR ITS QUICK RISE IN POPULARITY.

STEAKS

- ⅓ cup fresh lime juice
- ¼ cup extra virgin olive oil
- ¼ cup coarsely chopped cilantro
- 5 cloves garlic, minced
- 4 6-ounce flat-iron (boneless beef shoulder top blade) steaks

SALSA SALAD

- 1 seedless (English) cucumber (peeled if desired), diced
- 1 cup quartered grape tomatoes
- ½ cup diced red onion
- ½ cup coarsely chopped cilantro
- 1 poblano chile, seeded and diced (see tip)
- 1 jalapeño, seeded and minced (see tip)
- 3 tablespoons fresh lime juice
- 2 tablespoons extra virgin olive oil

CARAMELIZED ONIONS

- 2 tablespoons extra virgin olive oil
- 2 large sweet onions (such as Maui, Vidalia, Texas Sweet, or Walla Walla)

½ teaspoon ground chipotle chile pepper

1. For steaks, place steaks in a resealable plastic bag set in a shallow dish; set aside. In a small bowl combine lime juice, oil, cilantro, and garlic; pour over steaks in bag. Seal bag; turn to coat. Marinate in the refrigerator for 2 hours.

2. For salad, in a large bowl combine cucumber, tomatoes, onion, cilantro, poblano, and jalapeño. Toss to combine. For dressing, in a small bowl whisk together lime juice and olive oil together. Drizzle dressing over vegetables; toss to coat. Cover and refrigerate until serving time.

3. For onions, preheat oven to 400°F. Brush the inside of a Dutch oven with some of the olive oil; set aside. Cut onions in half lengthwise, remove skins, and then slice crosswise ¼ inch thick. In the Dutch oven combine the remaining olive oil, the onions, and the chipotle chile pepper. Cover and bake for 20 minutes. Uncover and let cool about 20 minutes.

4. Transfer cooled onions to a foil grilling bag or wrap onions in a double thickness of foil. Puncture the top of the foil in several places with a skewer.

5. For a charcoal grill, arrange medium-hot coals around perimeter of grill. Test for medium heat above center of grill. Place packet in center of grill rack. Cover and grill about 45 minutes or until onions are soft and amber color. (For a gas grill, preheat grill. Reduce heat to medium. Adjust for indirect cooking. Place packet over the burner that is turned off. Cover and grill as directed.)

6. Remove steaks from marinade; discard marinade. For a charcoal or gas grill, place steaks on the grill rack directly over medium-high heat. Cover and grill for 8 to 10 minutes or until an instant-read thermometer inserted horizontally into the steaks reads 135°F, turning once. Transfer steaks to a platter, cover loosely with foil and let stand for 10 minutes.

7. To serve, divide salsa salad among four serving plates. Place a steak on each plate and top with a mound of caramelized onions. Serve immediately.

Make-Ahead Directions: Salsa salad may be made and refrigerated up to 4 hours before serving.

GRILLED RIBEYES WITH HERBED ONION AND GARLIC "BUTTER"

PREP: 10 minutes COOK: 12 minutes CHILL: 30 minutes GRILL: 11 minutes MAKES: 4 servings

THE HEAT FROM JUST-OFF-THE-GRILL STEAKS MELTS THE MOUNDS OF CARAMELIZED ONIONS, GARLIC, AND HERBS SUSPENDED IN A RICH-TASTING BLEND OF COCONUT OIL AND OLIVE OIL.

2 tablespoons unrefined coconut oil

1 small onion, halved and cut into very thin slivers (about ¾ cup)

1 clove garlic, very thinly sliced

2 tablespoons extra virgin olive oil

1 tablespoon snipped fresh parsley

2 teaspoons snipped fresh thyme, rosemary, and/or oregano

4 8- to 10-ounce beef ribeye steaks, cut 1 inch thick

½ teaspoon freshly ground black pepper

1. In a medium skillet melt coconut oil over low heat. Add onion; cook for 10 to 15 minutes or until lightly browned, stirring occasionally. Add garlic; cook for 2 to 3 minutes more or until onion is golden brown, stirring occasionally.

2. Transfer onion mixture to a small bowl. Stir in olive oil, parsley, and thyme. Refrigerate, uncovered, for 30 minutes or until mixture is firm enough to mound when scooped, stirring occasionally.

3. Meanwhile, sprinkle steaks with pepper. For a charcoal or gas grill, place steaks on the grill rack directly over medium heat. Cover and grill for 11 to 15 minutes for

medium rare (145°F) or 14 to 18 minutes for medium (160°F), turning once halfway through grilling.

4. To serve, place each steak on a serving plate. Immediately scoop onion mixture evenly onto steaks.

RIBEYE SALAD WITH GRILLED BEETS

PREP: 20 minutes GRILL: 55 minutes STAND: 5 minutes MAKES: 4 servings

THE EARTHY FLAVOR OF BEETS PAIRS BEAUTIFULLY WITH THE SWEETNESS OF THE ORANGES—AND THE TOASTED PECANS ADD A BIT OF CRUNCH TO THIS MAIN-DISH SALAD THAT'S PERFECT FOR EATING OUTDOORS ON A WARM SUMMER NIGHT.

1 pound medium golden and/or red beets, scrubbed, trimmed, and cut into wedges
1 small onion, cut into thin wedges
2 sprigs fresh thyme
1 tablespoon extra virgin olive oil
Cracked black pepper
2 8-ounce boneless beef ribeye steaks, cut ¾ inch thick
2 cloves garlic, halved
2 tablespoons Mediterranean Seasoning (see recipe)
6 cups mixed greens
2 oranges, peeled, sectioned, and coarsely chopped
½ cup chopped pecans, toasted (see tip)
½ cup Bright Citrus Vinaigrette (see recipe)

1. Place beets, onion, and thyme sprigs in a foil pan. Drizzle with oil and toss to combine; sprinkle lightly with cracked black pepper. For a charcoal or gas grill, place pan on the center of the grill rack. Cover and grill 55 to 60 minutes or until tender when pierced with a knife, stirring occasionally.

2. Meanwhile, rub both sides of the steaks with cut sides of garlic; sprinkle with Mediterranean Seasoning.

3. Move beets from center of grill to make room for steaks. Add steaks to grill directly over medium heat. Cover and

grill for 11 to 15 minutes for medium rare (145°F) or 14 to 18 minutes for medium (160°F), turning once halfway through grilling. Remove foil pan and steaks from grill. Let steaks stand for 5 minutes. Discard thyme sprigs from foil pan.

4. Thinly slice steak diagonally into bite-size pieces. Divide greens among four serving plates. Top with sliced steak, beets, onion wedges, chopped oranges, and pecans. Drizzle with Bright Citrus Vinaigrette.

KOREAN-STYLE SHORT RIBS WITH SAUTÉED GINGER CABBAGE

PREP: 50 minutes COOK: 25 minutes BAKE: 10 hours CHILL: overnight MAKES: 4 servings

MAKE SURE THE LID OF YOUR DUTCH OVEN FITS VERY TIGHTLY SO THAT DURING THE VERY LONG BRAISING TIME, THE COOKING LIQUID DOESN'T ALL EVAPORATE THROUGH A GAP BETWEEN THE LID AND POT.

1 ounce dried shiitake mushrooms
1½ cups sliced scallions
1 Asian pear, peeled, cored, and chopped
1 3-inch piece fresh ginger, peeled and chopped
1 serrano chile pepper, finely chopped (seeded if desired) (see tip)
5 cloves garlic
1 tablespoon refined coconut oil
5 pounds bone-in beef short ribs
Freshly ground black pepper
4 cups Beef Bone Broth (see recipe) or no-salt-added beef broth
2 cups sliced fresh shiitake mushrooms
1 tablespoon finely shredded orange peel
⅓ cup fresh juice
Sautéed Ginger Cabbage (see recipe, below)
Finely shredded orange peel (optional)

1. Preheat oven to 325°F. Place dried shiitake mushrooms in a small bowl; add enough boiling water to cover. Let stand about 30 minutes or until rehydrated and soft. Drain, reserving the soaking liquid. Finely chop the mushrooms. Place mushrooms in a small bowl; cover and refrigerate until needed in Step 4. Set mushrooms and liquid aside.

2. For sauce, in a food processor combine scallions, Asian pear, ginger, serrano, garlic, and the reserved mushroom soaking liquid. Cover and process until smooth. Set sauce aside.

3. In a 6-quart Dutch oven heat the coconut oil over medium-high heat. Sprinkle short ribs with freshly ground black pepper. Cook ribs, in batches, in hot coconut oil about 10 minutes or until well browned on all sides, turning halfway through cooking. Return all the ribs to the pot; add sauce and Beef Bone broth. Cover the Dutch oven with a tight-fitting lid. Bake about 10 hours or until meat is very tender and falls off the bones.

4. Carefully remove the ribs from sauce. Place ribs and sauce in separate containers. Cover and refrigerate overnight. When cold, remove fat from surface of the sauce and discard. Bring the sauce to boiling over high heat; add hydrated mushrooms from Step 1 and the fresh mushrooms. Boil gently for 10 minutes to reduce sauce and intensify flavors. Return ribs to the sauce; simmer until heated through. Stir in 1 tablespoon orange peel and the orange juice. Serve with Sautéed Ginger Cabbage. If desired, sprinkle with additional orange peel.

Sautéed Ginger Cabbage: In a large skillet heat 1 tablespoon refined coconut oil over medium-high heat. Add 2 tablespoons minced fresh ginger; 2 cloves garlic, minced; and crushed red pepper to taste. Cook and stir until fragrant, about 30 seconds. Add 6 cups shredded napa, savoy, or green cabbage and 1 Asian pear, peeled, cored, and thinly sliced. Cook and stir for 3 minutes or until cabbage wilts slightly and pear softens. Stir in ½ cup unsweetened apple juice. Cover and cook about 2 minutes until cabbage is tender. Stir in ½ cup sliced scallions and 1 tablespoon sesame seeds.

BEEF SHORT RIBS WITH CITRUS-FENNEL GREMOLATA

PREP: 40 minutes GRILL: 8 minutes SLOW COOK: 9 hours (low) or 4½ hours (high) MAKES: 4 servings

GREMOLATA IS A FLAVORFUL BLEND OF PARSLEY, GARLIC, AND LEMON PEEL THAT IS SPRINKLED ON OSSO BUCCO—THE CLASSIC ITALIAN DISH OF BRAISED VEAL SHANKS—TO BRIGHTEN ITS RICH, UNCTUOUS FLAVOR. WITH THE ADDITION OF ORANGE PEEL AND FRESH FEATHERY FENNEL FRONDS, IT DOES THE SAME FOR THESE TENDER BEEF SHORT RIBS.

RIBS
- 2½ to 3 pounds bone-in beef short ribs
- 3 tablespoons Lemon-Herb Seasoning (see recipe)
- 1 medium fennel bulb
- 1 large onion, cut into large wedges
- 2 cups Beef Bone Broth (see recipe) or no-salt-added beef broth
- 2 cloves garlic, halved

PAN-ROASTED SQUASH
- 3 tablespoons extra virgin olive oil
- 1 pound butternut squash, peeled, seeded, and cut into ½-inch pieces (about 2 cups)
- 4 teaspoons snipped fresh thyme
- Extra virgin olive oil

GREMOLATA
- ¼ cup snipped fresh parsley
- 2 tablespoons minced garlic
- 1½ teaspoons finely shredded lemon peel
- 1½ teaspoons finely shredded orange peel

1. Sprinkle short ribs with Lemon-Herb Seasoning; lightly rub into meat with your fingers; set aside. Remove fronds from fennel; set aside for Citrus-Fennel Gremolata. Trim and quarter fennel bulb.

2. For a charcoal grill, arrange medium-hot coals on one side of the grill. Test for medium heat above the side of grill without coals. Place short ribs on grill rack on side without coals; place fennel quarters and onion wedges on the rack directly over coals. Cover and grill for 8 to 10 minutes or until vegetables and ribs are just browned, turning once halfway through grilling. (For a gas grill, preheat grill, reduce heat to medium. Adjust for indirect cooking. Place ribs on grill rack over burner that is turned off; place fennel and onion on rack over burner that is turned on. Cover and grill as directed.) When cool enough to handle, coarsely chop the fennel and onion.

3. In a 5- to 6-quart slow cooker combine chopped fennel and onion, Beef Bone Broth, and garlic. Add ribs. Cover and cook on low-heat setting for 9 to 10 hours or 4½ to 5 hours on high-heat setting. Using a slotted spoon, transfer ribs to a platter; cover with foil to keep warm.

4. Meanwhile, for the squash, in a large skillet heat the 3 tablespoons oil over medium-high heat. Add squash and 3 teaspoons of the thyme, stirring to coat the squash. Arrange squash in a single layer in skillet and cook without stirring about 3 minutes or until browned on bottom sides. Turn squash pieces over; cook about 3 minutes more or until second sides are browned. Reduce heat to low; cover and cook for 10 to 15 minutes or until

tender. Sprinkle with remaining 1 teaspoon fresh thyme; drizzle with additional extra virgin olive oil.

5. For the gremolata, finely chop enough reserved fennel fronds to make ¼ cup. In a small bowl stir together the chopped fennel fronds, parsley, garlic, lemon peel, and orange peel.

6. Sprinkle gremolata over ribs. Serve with squash.

SWEDISH-STYLE BEEF PATTIES WITH MUSTARD-DILL CUCUMBER SALAD

PREP: 30 minutes COOK: 15 minutes MAKES: 4 servings

BEEF À LA LINDSTROM IS A SWEDISH HAMBURGER THAT IS TRADITIONALLY STUDDED WITH ONIONS, CAPERS, AND PICKLED BEETS SERVED WITH GRAVY AND WITHOUT A BUN. THIS ALLSPICE-INFUSED VERSION SUBSTITUTES ROASTED BEETS FOR THE SALT-LADEN PICKLED BEETS AND CAPERS AND IS TOPPED WITH A FRIED EGG.

CUCUMBER SALAD
- 2 teaspoons fresh orange juice
- 2 teaspoons white wine vinegar
- 1 teaspoon Dijon-Style Mustard (see recipe)
- 1 tablespoon extra virgin olive oil
- 1 large seedless (English) cucumber, peeled and sliced
- 2 tablespoons sliced scallions
- 1 tablespoon chopped fresh dill

BEEF PATTIES
- 1 pound ground beef
- ¼ cup finely chopped onion
- 1 tablespoon Dijon-Style Mustard (see recipe)
- ¾ teaspoon black pepper
- ½ teaspoon ground allspice
- ½ of a small beet, roasted, peeled, and finely diced*
- 2 tablespoons extra virgin olive oil
- ½ cup Beef Bone Broth (see recipe) or no-salt-added beef broth
- 4 large eggs
- 1 tablespoon finely chopped chives

1. For cucumber salad, in a large bowl whisk together orange juice, vinegar, and Dijon-Style Mustard. Slowly add olive oil in a thin stream, whisking until dressing thickens slightly. Add cucumber, scallions, and dill; toss until combined. Cover and refrigerate until serving time.

2. For beef patties, in a large bowl combine ground beef, onion, Dijon-Style Mustard, pepper, and allspice. Add roasted beet and gently mix until evenly incorporated into the meat. Shape mixture into four ½-inch-thick patties.

3. In a large skillet heat 1 tablespoon olive oil over medium-high heat. Fry patties about 8 minutes or until browned on the exterior and cooked through (160°), turning once. Transfer patties to a plate and cover loosely with foil to keep warm. Add Beef Bone Broth, stirring to scrape up browned bits from bottom of skillet. Cook about 4 minutes or until reduced by half. Drizzle patties with reduced pan juices and re-cover loosely.

4. Rinse and wipe out skillet with a paper towel. Heat the remaining 1 tablespoon olive oil over medium heat. Fry eggs in hot oil for 3 to 4 minutes or until whites are cooked but yolks remain soft and runny.

5. Place an egg on each beef patty. Sprinkle with chives and serve with cucumber salad.

*Tip: To roast beet, scrub well and place on a piece of aluminum foil. Drizzle with a little olive oil. Wrap in foil and seal tightly. Roast in a 375°F oven about 30 minutes or until a fork easily pierces beet. Let cool; slip skin off.

(Beet can be roasted up to 3 days ahead. Tightly wrap peeled roasted beets and store in the refrigerator.)

SMOTHERED BEEFBURGERS ON ARUGULA WITH ROASTED ROOT VEGETABLES

PREP: 40 minutes COOK: 35 minutes ROAST: 20 minutes MAKES: 4 servings

THERE ARE A LOT OF ELEMENTS TO THESE HEARTY BURGERS—AND THEY DO TAKE A BIT OF TIME TO PUT TOGETHER—BUT THE INCREDIBLE COMBINATION OF FLAVORS MAKES IT WELL WORTH THE EFFORT: A MEATY BURGER IS TOPPED WITH CARAMELIZED ONION AND MUSHROOM PAN SAUCE AND SERVED WITH SWEET ROASTED VEGETABLES AND PEPPERY ARUGULA.

- 5 tablespoons extra virgin olive oil
- 2 cups sliced fresh button, cremini, and/or shiitake mushrooms
- 3 yellow onions, thinly sliced*
- 2 teaspoons caraway seeds
- 3 carrots, peeled and cut into 1-inch chunks
- 2 parsnips, peeled and cut into 1-inch chunks
- 1 acorn squash, halved, seeded, and cut into wedges
- Freshly ground black pepper
- 2 pounds ground beef
- ½ cup finely chopped onion
- 1 tablespoon salt-free all-purpose seasoning blend
- 2 cups Beef Bone Broth (see recipe) or no-salt-added beef broth
- ¼ cup unsweetened apple juice
- 1 to 2 tablespoons dry sherry or white wine vinegar
- 1 tablespoon Dijon-Style Mustard (see recipe)
- 1 tablespoon snipped fresh thyme leaves
- 1 tablespoon snipped fresh parsley leaves
- 8 cups arugula leaves

1. Preheat oven to 425°F. For sauce, in a large skillet heat 1 tablespoon of the olive oil over medium-high heat. Add mushrooms; cook and stir about 8 minutes or until well browned and tender. Using a slotted spoon, transfer the mushrooms to a plate. Return the skillet to the burner; reduce heat to medium. Add the remaining 1 tablespoon olive oil, sliced onions, and the caraway seeds. Cover and cook for 20 to 25 minutes or until onions are very soft and richly browned, stirring occasionally. (Adjust heat as needed to prevent the onions from burning.)

2. Meanwhile, for roasted root vegetables, on a large baking sheet arrange carrots, parsnips, and squash. Drizzle with 2 tablespoons olive oil and sprinkle with pepper to taste; toss to coat vegetables. Roast for 20 to 25 minutes or until tender and beginning to brown, turning once halfway through roasting. Keep vegetables warm until ready to serve.

3. For burgers, in a large bowl combine the ground beef, finely chopped onion, and seasoning blend. Divide meat mixture into four equal portions and shape into patties, about ¾ inch thick. In an extra-large skillet heat the remaining 1 tablespoon olive oil over medium-high heat. Add burgers to skillet; cook about 8 minutes or until seared on both sides, turning once. Transfer burgers to a plate.

4. Add caramelized onions, reserved mushrooms, Beef Bone Broth, apple juice, sherry, and Dijon-Style Mustard to the skillet, stirring to combine. Return burgers to skillet. Bring to simmering. Cook until burgers are done (160°F), about

7 to 8 minutes. Stir in fresh thyme, parsley, and pepper to taste.

5. To serve, arrange 2 cups of arugula on each of four serving plates. Divide the roasted vegetables among the salads, then top with burgers. Generously spoon the onion mixture on the burgers.

*Tip: A mandoline slicer is a great help in thinly slicing onions.

GRILLED BEEFBURGERS WITH SESAME-CRUSTED TOMATOES

PREP: 30 minutes STAND: 20 minutes GRILL: 10 minutes MAKES: 4 servings

CRISP, GOLDEN-BROWN SESAME-CRUSTED SLICES OF TOMATO STAND IN FOR THE TRADITIONAL SESAME SEED BUN IN THESE SMOKY BURGERS. SERVE THEM WITH A KNIFE AND FORK.

4 ½-inch-thick red or green tomato slices*
1¼ pounds lean ground beef
1 tablespoon Smoky Seasoning (see recipe)
1 large egg
¾ cup almond meal
¼ cup sesame seeds
¼ teaspoon black pepper
1 small red onion, halved and sliced
1 tablespoon extra virgin olive oil
¼ cup refined coconut oil
1 small head Bibb lettuce
Paleo Ketchup (see recipe)
Dijon-Style Mustard (see recipe)

1. Place tomato slices on a double layer of paper towels. Top tomatoes with another double layer of paper towels. Press down lightly on paper towels so they stick to the tomatoes. Let stand at room temperature for 20 to 30 minutes so some of the tomato juice is absorbed.

2. Meanwhile, in a large bowl combine ground beef and Smoky Seasoning. Shape into four ½-inch-thick patties.

3. In a shallow bowl lightly beat egg with a fork. In another shallow bowl combine almond meal, sesame seeds, and

pepper. Dip each tomato slice into the egg, turning to coat. Allow excess egg to drip off. Dip each tomato slice into almond meal mixture, turning to coat. Place coated tomatoes on a flat plate; set aside. Toss onion slices with olive oil; place onion slices in a grill basket.

4. For a charcoal or gas grill, place onions in basket and beef patties on grill rack over medium heat. Cover and grill for 10 to 12 minutes or onions are golden brown and lightly charred and patties are done (160°), stirring onions occasionally and turning patties once.

5. Meanwhile, in a large skillet heat oil over medium heat. Add tomato slices; cook for 8 to 10 minutes or until golden brown, turning once. (If tomatoes brown too quickly, reduce heat to medium-low. If necessary, add additional oil.) Drain on a paper towel-lined plate.

6. To serve, divide lettuce among four serving plates. Top with patties, onions, Paleo Ketchup, Dijon-Style Mustard, and sesame-crusted tomatoes.

*Note: You'll probably need 2 large tomatoes. If using red tomatoes, choose tomatoes that are just ripe but still slightly firm.

BURGERS ON A STICK WITH BABA GHANOUSH DIPPING SAUCE

SOAK: 15 minutes PREP: 20 minutes GRILL: 35 minutes MAKES: 4 servings

BABA GHANOUSH IS A MIDDLE EASTERN SPREAD MADE FROM SMOKY GRILLED EGGPLANT PUREED WITH OLIVE OIL, LEMON, GARLIC, AND TAHINI, A PASTE MADE FROM GROUND SESAME SEEDS. A SPRINKLING OF SESAME SEEDS IS FINE, BUT WHEN THEY ARE MADE INTO OIL OR PASTE, THEY BECOME A CONCENTRATED SOURCE OF LINOLEIC ACID, WHICH CAN CONTRIBUTE TO INFLAMMATION. THE PINE NUT BUTTER USED HERE MAKES A FINE SUBSTITUTE.

4 dried tomatoes

1½ pounds lean ground beef

3 to 4 tablespoons finely chopped onion

1 tablespoon finely snipped fresh oregano and/or finely snipped fresh mint or ½ teaspoon dried oregano, crushed

¼ teaspoon cayenne pepper

Baba Ghanoush Dipping Sauce (see recipe, below)

1. Soak eight 10-inch wooden skewers in water for 30 minutes. Meanwhile, in a small bowl pour boiling water over tomatoes; let stand for 5 minutes to rehydrate. Drain tomatoes and pat dry with paper towels.

2. In large bowl combine chopped tomatoes, ground beef, onion, oregano, and cayenne pepper. Divide meat mixture into eight portions; roll each portion into a ball. Remove skewers from water; pat dry. Thread one ball onto a skewer and shape into a long oval around the skewer, starting just below the pointed tip and leaving enough

room on the other end to be able to hold the stick. Repeat with remaining skewers and balls.

3. For a charcoal or gas grill, place beef skewers on a grill rack directly over medium heat. Cover and grill about 6 minutes or until done (160°F), turning once halfway through grilling. Serve with Baba Ghanoush Dipping Sauce.

Baba Ghanoush Dipping Sauce: Poke 2 medium eggplants in several places with a fork. For a charcoal or gas grill, place eggplants on a grill rack directly over medium heat. Cover and grill for 10 minutes or until charred on all sides, turning several times during grilling. Remove eggplants and carefully wrap in foil. Place wrapped eggplants back on the grill rack but not directly over the coals. Cover and grill for 25 to 35 minutes more or until collapsed and very tender. Cool. Halve eggplants and scrape out the flesh; place flesh in a food processor. Add ¼ cup Pine Nut Butter (see recipe); ¼ cup fresh lemon juice; 2 cloves garlic, minced; 1 tablespoon extra virgin olive oil; 2 to 3 tablespoons snipped fresh parsley; and ½ teaspoon ground cumin. Cover and process just until almost smooth. If sauce is too thick for dipping, stir in enough water to make desired consistency.

SMOKY STUFFED SWEET PEPPERS

PREP: 20 minutes COOK: 8 minutes BAKE: 30 minutes MAKES: 4 servings

MAKE THIS FAMILY FAVORITE WITH A MIX OF COLORED SWEET PEPPERS FOR AN EYE-CATCHING DISH. THE FIRE-ROASTED TOMATOES ARE A FINE EXAMPLE OF HOW TO ADD GREAT TASTE TO FOOD IN A HEALTHY WAY. THE SIMPLE ACT OF SLIGHTLY CHARRING THE TOMATOES BEFORE THEY ARE CANNED (WITHOUT SALT) BUMPS UP THEIR FLAVOR.

- 4 large green, red, yellow, and/or orange sweet peppers
- 1 pound ground beef
- 1 tablespoon Smoky Seasoning (see recipe)
- 1 tablespoon extra virgin olive oil
- 1 small yellow onion, chopped
- 3 cloves garlic, minced
- 1 small head cauliflower, cored and broken into florets
- 1 15-ounce can no-salt-added diced fire-roasted tomatoes, drained
- ¼ cup finely chopped fresh parsley
- ½ teaspoon black pepper
- ⅛ teaspoon cayenne pepper
- ½ cup Walnut Crumb Topping (see recipe, below)

1. Preheat oven to 375°F. Cut sweet peppers in half vertically. Remove stems, seeds, and membranes; discard. Set pepper halves aside.

2. Place ground beef in a medium bowl; sprinkle with Smoky Seasoning. Use your hands to gently mix seasoning into meat.

3. In a large skillet heat olive oil over medium heat. Add meat, onion, and garlic; cook until meat is browned and onion is

tender, stirring with a wooden spoon to break up meat. Remove skillet from heat.

4. In a food processor process cauliflower florets until very finely chopped. (If you don't have a food processor, grate the cauliflower on a box grater.) Measure 3 cups of the cauliflower. Add to ground beef mixture in skillet. (If there is any remaining cauliflower, save it for another use.) Stir in drained tomatoes, parsley, black pepper, and cayenne pepper.

5. Fill pepper halves with ground beef mixture, packing it lightly and mounding slightly. Arrange filled pepper halves in a baking dish. Bake for 30 to 35 minutes or until peppers are crisp-tender.* Top with Walnut Crumb Topping. If desired, return to oven for 5 minutes to crisp topping before serving.

Walnut Crumb Topping: In a medium skillet heat 1 tablespoon extra virgin olive oil over medium low heat. Stir in 1 teaspoon dried thyme, 1 teaspoon smoked paprika, and ¼ teaspoon garlic powder. Add 1 cup very finely chopped walnuts. Cook and stir about 5 minutes or until walnuts are golden brown and lightly toasted. Stir in a dash or two of cayenne pepper. Let cool completely. Store leftover topping in a tightly sealed container in the refrigerator until ready to use. Makes 1 cup.

*Note: If using green peppers, bake for an additional 10 minutes.

BISON BURGERS WITH CABERNET ONIONS AND ARUGULA

PREP: 30 minutes COOK: 18 minutes GRILL: 10 minutes MAKES: 4 servings

BISON HAS A VERY LOW FAT CONTENT AND WILL COOK 30% TO 50% FASTER THAN BEEF. THE MEAT RETAINS ITS RED COLOR AFTER COOKING, SO COLOR IS NOT AN INDICATOR OF DONENESS. BECAUSE BISON IS SO LEAN, DO NOT COOK IT BEYOND AN INTERNAL TEMPERATURE OF 155°F.

  2 tablespoons extra virgin olive oil
  2 large sweet onions, thinly sliced
  ¾ cup Cabernet Sauvignon or other dry red wine
  1 teaspoon Mediterranean Seasoning (see recipe)
  ¼ cup extra virgin olive oil
  ¼ cup balsamic vinegar
  1 tablespoon finely chopped shallot
  1 tablespoon snipped fresh basil
  1 small clove garlic, minced
  1 pound ground bison
  ¼ cup Basil Pesto (see recipe)
  5 cups arugula
  Raw unsalted pistachios, toasted (see tip)

1. In a large skillet heat the 2 tablespoons oil over medium-low heat. Add onions. Cook, covered, for 10 to 15 minutes or until onions are tender, stirring occasionally. Uncover; cook and stir over medium-high heat for 3 to 5 minutes or until onions are golden. Add wine; cook about 5 minutes or until most of the wine evaporates. Sprinkle with Mediterranean Seasoning; keep warm.

2. Meanwhile, for vinaigrette, in a screw-top jar combine the ¼ cup olive oil, vinegar, shallot, basil, and garlic. Cover and shake well.

3. In a large bowl lightly mix ground bison and Basil Pesto. Lightly shape meat mixture into four ¾-inch-thick patties.

4. For a charcoal or gas grill, place patties on a lightly greased grill rack directly over medium heat. Cover and grill about 10 minutes to desired doneness (145°F for medium rare or 155°F for medium), turning once halfway through grilling.

5. Place arugula in a large bowl. Drizzle vinaigrette over arugula; toss to coat. To serve, divide onions among four serving plates; top each with a bison burger. Top burgers with arugula and sprinkle with pistachios.

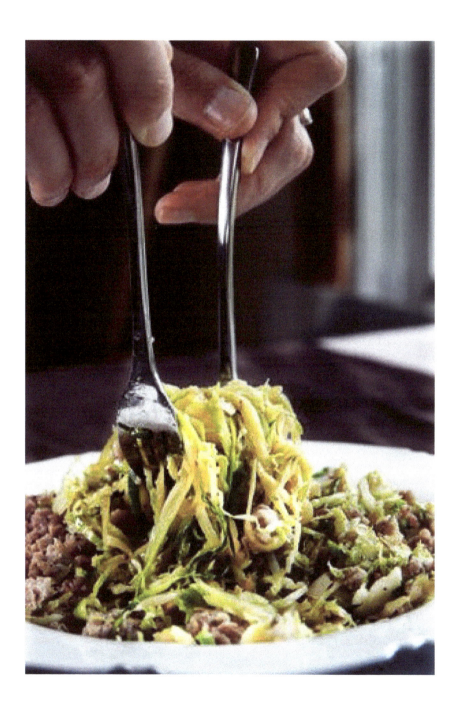

BISON AND LAMB MEAT LOAF ON CHARD AND SWEET POTATOES

PREP: 1 hour COOK: 20 minutes BAKE: 1 hour STAND: 10 minutes MAKES: 4 servings

THIS IS OLD-FASHIONED COMFORT FOOD WITH A MODERN TWIST. A RED-WINE PAN SAUCE GIVES THE MEAT LOAF A FLAVOR BOOST, AND THE GARLICKY CHARD AND SWEET POTATOES MASHED WITH CASHEW CREAM AND COCONUT OIL OFFER INCREDIBLE NUTRITIONAL CONTENT.

2 tablespoons olive oil
1 cup finely chopped cremini mushrooms
½ cup finely chopped red onion (1 medium)
½ cup finely chopped celery (1 stalk)
⅓ cup finely chopped carrot (1 small)
½ of a small apple, cored, peeled, and shredded
2 cloves garlic, minced
½ teaspoon Mediterranean Seasoning (see recipe)
1 large egg, lightly beaten
1 tablespoon snipped fresh sage
1 tablespoon snipped fresh thyme
8 ounces ground bison
8 ounces ground lamb or beef
¾ cup dry red wine
1 medium shallot, finely chopped
¾ cup Beef Bone Broth (see recipe) or no-salt-added beef broth
Mashed Sweet Potatoes (see recipe, below)
Garlicky Swiss Chard (see recipe, below)

1. Preheat oven to 350°F. In a large skillet heat oil over medium heat. Add mushrooms, onion, celery, and carrot; cook and stir about 5 minutes or until vegetables are

softened. Reduce heat to low; add shredded apple and garlic. Cook, covered, about 5 minutes or until vegetables are very tender. Remove from heat; stir in Mediterranean Seasoning.

2. Using a slotted spoon, transfer mushroom mixture to a large bowl, reserving drippings in skillet. Stir in egg, sage, and thyme. Add ground bison and ground lamb; lightly mix. Spoon meat mixture into a 2-quart rectangular baking dish; shape into a 7×4-inch rectangle. Bake about 1 hour or until an instant-read thermometer registers 155°F. Let stand for 10 minutes. Carefully remove meat loaf to a serving platter. Cover and keep warm.

3. For the pan sauce, scrape drippings and crusty browned bits from the baking dish into reserved drippings in the skillet. Add wine and shallot. Bring to boiling over medium heat; cook until reduced by half. Add Beef Bone Broth; cook and stir until reduced by half. Remove skillet from heat.

4. To serve, divide Mashed Sweet Potatoes among four serving plates; top with some of the Garlicky Swiss Chard. Slice meat loaf; place slices on Garlicky Swiss Chard and drizzle with the pan sauce.

Mashed Sweet Potatoes: Peel and coarsely chop 4 medium sweet potatoes. In a large saucepan cook potatoes in enough boiling water to cover for 15 minutes or until tender; drain. Mash with a potato masher. Add ½ cup Cashew Cream (see recipe) and 2 tablespoons unrefined coconut oil; mash until smooth. Keep warm.

Garlicky Swiss Chard: Remove stems from 2 bunches Swiss chard and discard. Coarsely chop leaves. In a large skillet heat 2 tablespoons olive oil over medium heat. Add Swiss chard and 2 cloves garlic, minced; cook until chard is wilted, tossing occasionally with tongs.

APPLE-CURRANT-SAUCED BISON MEATBALLS WITH ZUCCHINI PAPPARDELLE

PREP: 25 minutes BAKE: 15 minutes COOK: 18 minutes MAKES: 4 servings

THE MEATBALLS WILL BE VERY WET AS YOU FORM THEM. TO KEEP THE MEAT MIXTURE FROM STICKING TO YOUR HANDS, KEEP A BOWL OF COOL WATER HANDY AND WET YOUR HANDS OCCASIONALLY AS YOU WORK. CHANGE THE WATER A COUPLE OF TIMES AS YOU MAKE THE MEATBALLS.

MEATBALLS
- Olive oil
- ½ cup coarsely chopped red onion
- 2 cloves garlic, minced
- 1 egg, lightly beaten
- ½ cup finely chopped button mushrooms and stems
- 2 tablespoon snipped fresh Italian (flat-leaf) parsley
- 2 teaspoons olive oil
- 1 pound ground bison (coarse ground if available)

APPLE-CURRANT SAUCE
- 2 tablespoons olive oil
- 2 large Granny Smith apples, peeled, cored, and finely chopped
- 2 shallots, minced
- 2 tablespoons fresh lemon juice
- ½ cup Chicken Bone Broth (see recipe) or no-salt-added chicken broth
- 2 to 3 tablespoons dried currants

ZUCCHINI PAPPARDELLE
- 6 zucchini
- 2 tablespoons olive oil

¼ cup finely chopped scallions
½ teaspoon crushed red pepper
2 cloves garlic, minced

1. For meatballs, preheat oven to 375°F. Lightly brush a rimmed baking sheet with olive oil; set aside. In a food processor or blender combine onion and garlic. Pulse until smooth. Transfer onion mixture to a medium bowl. Add egg, mushrooms, parsley, and 2 teaspoons oil; stir to combine. Add ground bison; mix lightly but well. Divide meat mixture into 16 portions; shape into meatballs. Place meatballs, evenly spaced, on the prepared baking sheet. Bake for 15 minutes; set aside.

2. For sauce, in a skillet heat 2 tablespoons oil over medium heat. Add apples and shallots; cook and stir for 6 to 8 minutes or until very tender. Stir in lemon juice. Transfer mixture to a food processor or blender. Cover and process or blend until smooth; return to the skillet. Stir in Chicken Bone Broth and currants. Bring to boiling; reduce heat. Simmer, uncovered, for 8 to 10 minutes, stirring frequently. Add meatballs; cook and stir over low heat until heated through.

3. Meanwhile, for pappardelle, trim ends of zucchini. Using a mandoline or very sharp vegetable peeler, shave zucchini into thin ribbons. (To keep the ribbons intact, stop shaving once you reach the seeds in the center of the squash.) In a extra-large skillet heat 2 tablespoons oil over medium heat. Stir in scallions, crushed red pepper, and garlic; cook and stir for 30 seconds. Add zucchini ribbons. Cook and gently stir about 3 minutes or just until wilted.

4. To serve, divide pappardelle among four serving plates; top with meatballs and apple-currant sauce.

BISON-PORCINI BOLOGNESE WITH ROASTED GARLIC SPAGHETTI SQUASH

PREP: 30 minutes COOK: 1 hour 30 minutes BAKE: 35 minutes MAKES: 6 servings

IF YOU THOUGHT YOU'D EATEN YOUR LAST DISH OF SPAGHETTI WITH MEAT SAUCE WHEN YOU ADOPTED THE PALEO DIET®, THINK AGAIN. THIS RICH BOLOGNESE FLAVORED WITH GARLIC, RED WINE, AND EARTHY PORCINI MUSHROOMS IS LADELED OVER SWEET, TOOTHSOME STRANDS OF SPAGHETTI SQUASH. YOU WON'T MISS THE PASTA ONE BIT.

- 1 ounce dried porcini mushrooms
- 1 cup boiling water
- 3 tablespoons extra virgin olive oil
- 1 pound ground bison
- 1 cup finely chopped carrots (2)
- ½ cup chopped onion (1 medium)
- ½ cup finely chopped celery (1 stalk)
- 4 cloves garlic, minced
- 3 tablespoons salt-free tomato paste
- ½ cup red wine
- 2 15-ounce cans no-salt-added crushed tomatoes
- 1 teaspoon dried oregano, crushed
- 1 teaspoon dried thyme, crushed
- ½ teaspoon black pepper
- 1 medium spaghetti squash (2½ to 3 pounds)
- 1 bulb garlic

1. In a small bowl combine the porcini mushrooms and boiling water; let stand for 15 minutes. Strain through a sieve lined with 100%-cotton cheesecloth, reserving the soaking liquid. Chop the mushrooms; set side.

2. In a 4- to 5-quart Dutch oven heat 1 tablespoon of the olive oil over medium heat. Add ground bison, carrots, onion, celery, and garlic. Cook until meat is browned and vegetables are tender, stirring with a wooden spoon to break up meat. Add tomato paste; cook and stir for 1 minute. Add red wine; cook and stir for 1 minute. Stir in porcini mushrooms, tomatoes, oregano, thyme, and pepper. Add reserved mushroom liquid, being careful to avoid adding any sand or grit that may be present in the bottom of the bowl. Bring to boiling, stirring occasionally; reduce heat to low. Simmer, covered, for 1½ to 2 hours or until desired consistency.

3. Meanwhile, preheat oven to 375°F. Halve squash lengthwise; scrape out seeds. Place squash halves, cut sides down, in a large baking dish. Using a fork, prick the skin all over. Cut off the top ½ inch of the head of garlic. Place the garlic, cut end up, in the baking dish with the squash. Drizzle with the remaining 1 tablespoon olive oil. Bake for 35 to 45 minutes or until squash and garlic are tender.

4. Using a spoon and fork, remove and shred the squash flesh from each squash half; transfer to a bowl and cover to keep warm. When the garlic is cool enough to handle, squeeze the bulb from the bottom to pop out the cloves. Use a fork to mash the garlic cloves. Stir mashed garlic into the squash, distributing garlic evenly. To serve, spoon sauce over squash mixture.

BISON CHILI CON CARNE

PREP: 25 minutes COOK: 1 hour 10 minutes MAKES: 4 servings

UNSWEETENED CHOCOLATE, COFFEE, AND CINNAMON ADD INTEREST TO THIS HEARTY FAVORITE. IF YOU'D LIKE EVEN MORE SMOKY FLAVOR, SUBSTITUTE 1 TABLESPOON OF SWEET SMOKED PAPRIKA FOR THE REGULAR PAPRIKA.

- 3 tablespoons extra virgin olive oil
- 1 pound ground bison
- ½ cup chopped onion (1 medium)
- 2 cloves garlic, minced
- 2 14.5-ounce cans diced no-salt-added tomatoes, undrained
- 1 6-ounce can salt-free tomato paste
- 1 cup Beef Bone Broth (see recipe) or no-salt-added beef broth
- ½ cup strong coffee
- 2 ounces 99% cacao baking bar, chopped
- 1 tablespoon paprika
- 1 teaspoon ground cumin
- 1 teaspoon dried oregano
- 1½ teaspoons Smoky Seasoning (see recipe)
- ½ teaspoon ground cinnamon
- ⅓ cup pepitas
- 1 teaspoon olive oil
- ½ cup Cashew Cream (see recipe)
- 1 teaspoon fresh lime juice
- ½ cup fresh cilantro leaves
- 4 lime wedges

1. In a Dutch oven heat the 3 tablespoons olive oil over medium heat. Add ground bison, onion, and garlic; cook about 5 minutes or until meat is browned, stirring with a wooden spoon to break up meat. Stir in undrained

tomatoes, tomato paste, Beef Bone Broth, coffee, baking chocolate, paprika, cumin, oregano, 1 teaspoon of the Smoky Seasoning, and cinnamon. Bring to boiling; reduce heat. Simmer, covered, for 1 hour, stirring occasionally.

2. Meanwhile, in a small skillet toast pepitas in the 1 teaspoon olive oil over medium heat until they start to pop and turn golden. Place pepitas in a small bowl; add the remaining ½ teaspoon Smoky Seasoning; toss to coat.

3. In a small bowl combine Cashew Cream and lime juice.

4. To serve, ladle chili into bowls. Top servings with Cashew Cream, pepitas, and cilantro. Serve with lime wedges.

MOROCCAN-SPICED BISON STEAKS WITH GRILLED LEMONS

PREP: 10 minutes GRILL: 10 minutes MAKES: 4 servings

SERVE THESE QUICK-TO-FIX STEAKS WITH COOL AND CRISP SPICED CARROT SLAW (SEE RECIPE). IF YOU'RE CRAVING A TREAT, GRILLED PINEAPPLE WITH COCONUT CREAM (SEE RECIPE) WOULD BE A GREAT WAY TO END THE MEAL.

2 tablespoons ground cinnamon

2 tablespoons paprika

1 tablespoon garlic powder

¼ teaspoon cayenne pepper

4 6-ounce bison filet mignon steaks, cut ¾ to 1 inch thick

2 lemons, halved horizontally

1. In a small bowl stir together the cinnamon, paprika, garlic powder, and cayenne pepper. Pat steaks dry with paper towels. Rub both sides of steaks with the spice mixture.

2. For a charcoal or gas grill, place steaks on the grill rack directly over medium heat. Cover and grill for 10 to 12 minutes for medium rare (145°F) or 12 to 15 minutes for medium (155°F), turning once halfway through grilling. Meanwhile, place lemon halves, cut sides down, on grill rack. Grill for 2 to 3 minutes or until slightly charred and juicy.

3. Serve with grilled lemon halves to squeeze over steaks.

HERBES DE PROVENCE-RUBBED BISON SIRLOIN ROAST

PREP: 15 minutes COOK: 15 minutes ROAST: 1 hour 15 minutes STAND: 15 minutes
MAKES: 4 servings

HERBES DE PROVENCE IS A BLEND OF DRIED HERBS THAT GROW IN PROFUSION IN THE SOUTH OF FRANCE. THE MIX USUALLY CONTAINS SOME COMBINATION OF BASIL, FENNEL SEEDS, LAVENDER, MARJORAM, ROSEMARY, SAGE, SUMMER SAVORY, AND THYME. IT FLAVORS THIS VERY AMERICAN ROAST BEAUTIFULLY.

- 1 3-pound bison sirloin roast
- 3 tablespoons herbes de Provence
- 4 tablespoons extra virgin olive oil
- 3 cloves garlic, minced
- 4 small parsnips, peeled and chopped
- 2 ripe pears, cored and chopped
- ½ cup unsweetened pear nectar
- 1 to 2 teaspoons fresh thyme

1. Preheat oven to 375°F. Trim fat from roast. In a small bowl combine Herbes de Provence, 2 tablespoons of the olive oil, and garlic; rub over the entire roast.

2. Place the roast on a rack in a shallow roasting pan. Insert an oven-going thermometer into the center of the roast.* Roast, uncovered, for 15 minutes. Reduce oven temperature to 300°F. Roast for 60 to 65 minutes more or until meat thermometer registers 140°F (medium rare). Cover with foil and let stand for 15 minutes.

3. Meanwhile, in a large skillet heat the remaining 2 tablespoons olive oil over medium heat. Add parsnips and pears; cook for 10 minutes or until parsnips are crisp-tender, stirring occasionally. Add pear nectar; cook about 5 minutes or until sauce is slightly thickened. Sprinkle with thyme.

4. Thinly slice roast across the grain. Serve meat with parsnips and pears.

*Tip: Bison is very lean and cooks faster than beef. Additionally, the color of the meat is redder than beef, so you can't rely on a visual cue to determine doneness. You will need a meat thermometer to let you know when the meat is done. An oven-going thermometer is ideal, though not a necessity.

COFFEE-BRAISED BISON SHORT RIBS WITH TANGERINE GREMOLATA AND CELERY ROOT MASH

PREP: 15 minutes COOK: 2 hours 45 minutes MAKES: 6 servings

BISON SHORT RIBS ARE BIG AND MEATY. THEY REQUIRE A GOOD LONG COOK IN LIQUID TO GET TENDER. GREMOLATA MADE WITH TANGERINE PEEL BRIGHTENS UP THE FLAVOR OF THIS HEARTY DISH.

MARINADE
- 2 cups water
- 3 cups strong coffee, chilled
- 2 cups fresh tangerine juice
- 2 tablespoons snipped fresh rosemary
- 1 teaspoon coarsely ground black pepper
- 4 pounds bison short ribs, cut between ribs to separate

BRAISE
- 2 tablespoons olive oil
- 1 teaspoon black pepper
- 2 cups chopped onions
- ½ cup chopped shallots
- 6 garlic cloves, chopped
- 1 jalapeño chile, seeded and chopped (see tip)
- 1 cup strong coffee
- 1 cup Beef Bone Broth (see recipe) or no-salt-added beef broth
- ¼ cup Paleo Ketchup (see recipe)
- 2 tablespoons Dijon-Style Mustard (see recipe)
- 3 tablespoons cider vinegar
- Celery Root Mash (see recipe, below)
- Tangerine Gremolata (see recipe, right)

1. For the marinade, in a large nonreactive container (glass or stainless steel) combine water, chilled coffee, tangerine juice, rosemary, and black pepper. Add ribs. Place a plate on top of ribs if necessary to keep them submerged. Cover and chill 4 to 6 hours, rearranging and stirring once.

2. For the braise, preheat oven to 325°F. Drain ribs, discarding marinade. Pat ribs dry with paper towels. In a large Dutch oven heat olive oil over medium-high heat. Season ribs with black pepper. Brown ribs in batches until browned on all sides, about 5 minutes per batch. Transfer to a large plate.

3. Add onions, shallots, garlic, and jalapeño to pot. Reduce heat to medium, cover, and cook until vegetables are soft, stirring occasionally, about 10 minutes. Add coffee and broth; stir, scraping up browned bits. Add Paleo Ketchup, Dijon-Style Mustard, and vinegar. Bring to boiling. Add ribs. Cover and transfer to oven. Cook until meat is tender, about 2 hours 15 minutes, stirring gently and rearranging ribs once or twice.

4. Transfer ribs to a plate; tent with foil to keep warm. Spoon fat from surface of sauce. Boil sauce until reduced to 2 cups, about 5 minutes. Divide Celery Root Mash among 6 plates; top with ribs and sauce. Sprinkle with Tangerine Gremolata.

Celery Root Mash: In a large saucepan combine 3 pounds celery root, peeled and cut into 1-inch pieces and 4 cups Chicken Bone Broth (see recipe) or unsalted chicken broth. Bring to boiling; reduce heat. Drain celery root, reserving broth. Return celery root to saucepan. Add 1 tablespoon olive oil and 2 teaspoons snipped fresh thyme. Using a potato masher, mash the celery root, adding reserved broth, a few tablespoons at a time, as needed to achieve desired consistency.

Tangerine Gremolata: In a small bowl combine ½ cup snipped fresh parsley, 2 tablespoons finely shredded tangerine peel, and 2 cloves minced garlic.

BEEF BONE BROTH

PREP: 25 minutes **ROAST:** 1 hour **COOK:** 8 hours **MAKES:** 8 to 10 cups

BONY OXTAILS MAKE AN EXTREMELY RICH-TASTING BROTH THAT CAN BE USED IN ANY RECIPE THAT CALLS FOR BEEF BROTH—OR SIMPLY ENJOYED AS A PICK-ME-UP IN A MUG ANY TIME OF DAY. THOUGH THEY ACTUALLY USED TO COME FROM AN OX, OXTAILS NOW COME FROM A BEEF ANIMAL.

- 5 carrots, roughly chopped
- 5 stalks celery, roughly chopped
- 2 yellow onions, unpeeled, halved
- 8 ounces white mushrooms
- 1 bulb garlic, unpeeled, halved
- 2 pounds oxtail bones or beef bones
- 2 tomatoes
- 12 cups cold water
- 3 bay leaves

1. Preheat oven to 400°F. In a large rimmed baking sheet or shallow baking pan arrange the carrots, celery, onions, mushrooms, and garlic; place the bones on top of the vegetables. In a food processor pulse tomatoes until smooth. Spread tomatoes over the bones to coat (it's okay if some of the puree drips onto the pan and the vegetables). Roast for 1 to 1½ hours or until bones are deep brown and the vegetables are caramelized. Transfer bones and vegetables to a 10- to 12-quart Dutch oven or stockpot. (If some of the tomato mixture caramelizes on the bottom of the pan, add 1 cup of hot water to the pan and scrape up any bits. Pour the liquid over the bones and

vegetables and reduce water amount by 1 cup.) Add the cold water and bay leaves.

2. Slowly bring the mixture to a simmer over medium-high to high heat. Reduce heat; cover and simmer broth for 8 to 10 hours, stirring occasionally.

3. Strain broth; discard bones and vegetables. Cool broth; transfer broth to storage containers and refrigerate for up to 5 days; freeze for up to 3 months.*

Slow Cooker Directions: For a 6- to 8-quart slow cooker, use 1 pound beef bones, 3 carrots, 3 stalks celery, 1 yellow onion, and 1 bulb garlic. Puree 1 tomato and rub onto the bones. Roast as directed, then transfer the bones and vegetables to the slow cooker. Scrape off any caramelized tomato as directed and add to the slow cooker. Add enough water to cover. Cover and cook on high-heat setting until broth comes to boiling, about 4 hours. Reduce to low-heat setting; cook for 12 to 24 hours. Strain broth; discard bones and vegetables. Store as directed.

*Tip: To easily skim fat off broth, store broth in a covered container in the refrigerator overnight. Fat will rise to the top and form a firm layer that can easily be scraped off. Broth may thicken after chilling.

TUNISIAN SPICE-RUBBED PORK SHOULDER WITH SPICY SWEET POTATO FRIES

PREP: 25 minutes ROAST: 4 hours BAKE: 30 minutes MAKES: 4 servings

THIS IS A GREAT DISH TO MAKE ON A COOL FALL DAY. THE MEAT ROASTS FOR HOURS IN THE OVEN, MAKING YOUR HOUSE SMELL WONDERFUL AND GIVING YOU TIME TO DO OTHER THINGS. OVEN-BAKED SWEET POTATO FRIES DON'T GET CRISP IN THE SAME WAY THAT WHITE POTATOES DO, BUT THEY ARE DELICIOUS IN THEIR OWN WAY, ESPECIALLY WHEN DIPPED IN GARLICKY MAYONNAISE.

PORK

- 1 2½- to 3-pound bone-in pork shoulder roast
- 2 teaspoons ground ancho chile pepper
- 2 teaspoons ground cumin
- 1 teaspoon caraway seeds, lightly crushed
- 1 teaspoon ground coriander
- ½ teaspoon ground turmeric
- ¼ teaspoon ground cinnamon
- 3 tablespoons olive oil

FRIES

- 4 medium sweet potatoes (about 2 pounds), peeled and cut into ½-inch-thick wedges
- ½ teaspoon crushed red pepper
- ½ teaspoon onion powder
- ½ teaspoon garlic powder
- Olive oil
- 1 onion, thinly sliced
- Paleo Aïoli (Garlic Mayo) (see recipe)

1. Preheat oven to 300°F. Trim fat from meat. In a small bowl combine ground ancho chile pepper, ground cumin, caraway seeds, coriander, turmeric, and cinnamon. Sprinkle meat with spice mixture; using your fingers, rub evenly into meat.

2. In an ovenproof 5- to 6-quart Dutch oven heat 1 tablespoon of the olive oil over medium-high heat. Brown pork on all sides in hot oil. Cover and roast about 4 hours or until very tender and meat thermometer registers 190°F. Remove Dutch oven from oven. Let stand, covered, while you prepare the sweet potato fries and the onions, reserving 1 tablespoon of the fat in the Dutch oven.

3. Increase oven temperature to 400°F. For the sweet potato fries, in a large bowl combine sweet potatoes, the remaining 2 tablespoons olive oil, crushed red pepper, onion powder, and garlic powder; toss to coat. Line one large or two small baking sheets with foil; brush with additional olive oil. Arrange sweet potatoes in a single layer on the prepared baking sheet(s). Bake about 30 minutes or until tender, turning the sweet potatoes once halfway through baking.

4. Meanwhile, remove meat from Dutch oven; cover with foil to keep warm. Drain drippings, reserving 1 tablespoon fat. Return the reserved fat to Dutch oven. Add onion; cook over medium heat about 5 minutes or until just softened, stirring occasionally.

5. Transfer the pork and onion to a serving platter. Using two forks, pull the pork into large shreds. Serve pork and fries with Paleo Aïoli.

CUBAN GRILLED PORK SHOULDER

PREP: 15 minutes MARINATE: 24 hours GRILL: 2 hours 30 minutes STAND: 10 minutes
MAKES: 6 to 8 servings

KNOWN AS "LECHON ASADO" IN ITS COUNTRY OF ORIGIN, THIS PORK ROAST IS MARINATED IN A COMBINATION OF FRESH CITRUS JUICES, SPICES, CRUSHED RED PEPPER, AND AN ENTIRE BULB OF MINCED GARLIC. COOKING IT OVER HOT COALS AFTER AN OVERNIGHT SOAK IN THE MARINADE INFUSES IT WITH AMAZING FLAVOR.

1 bulb garlic, cloves separated, peeled, and minced
1 cup coarsely chopped onions
1 cup olive oil
1⅓ cups fresh lime juice
⅔ cup fresh orange juice
1 tablespoon ground cumin
1 tablespoon dried oregano, crushed
2 teaspoons freshly ground black pepper
1 teaspoon crushed red pepper
1 4- to 5-pound boneless pork shoulder roast

1. For marinade, separate garlic head into cloves. Peel and mince cloves; place in a large bowl. Add onions, olive oil, lime juice, orange juice, cumin, oregano, black pepper, and crushed red pepper. Stir well and set aside.

2. Using a boning knife, deeply puncture pork roast all over. Carefully lower roast into the marinade, submerging it as much as possible in the liquid. Cover bowl tightly with plastic wrap. Marinate in the refrigerator for 24 hours, turning once.

3. Remove pork from marinade. Pour marinade into a medium saucepan. Bring to boiling; boil for 5 minutes. Remove from heat and let cool. Set aside.

4. For a charcoal grill, arrange medium-hot coals around a drip pan. Test for medium heat above the pan. Place meat on grill rack over drip pan. Cover and grill for 2½ to 3 hours or until an instant-read thermometer inserted into center of roast registers 140°F. (For a gas grill, preheat grill. Reduce heat to medium. Adjust for indirect cooking. Place meat on grill rack over burner that is turned off. Cover and grill as directed.) Remove meat from grill. Cover loosely with foil and let stand for 10 minutes before carving or pulling.

ITALIAN SPICE-RUBBED PORK ROAST WITH VEGETABLES

PREP: 20 minutes ROAST: 2 hours 25 minutes STAND: 10 minutes MAKES: 8 servings

"FRESH IS BEST" IS A GOOD MANTRA TO FOLLOW WHEN IT COMES TO COOKING MOST OF THE TIME. HOWEVER, DRIED HERBS WORK VERY WELL IN RUBS FOR MEATS. WHEN HERBS ARE DRIED, THEIR FLAVORS ARE CONCENTRATED. WHEN THEY COME INTO CONTACT WITH MOISTURE FROM THE MEAT, THEY RELEASE THEIR FLAVORS INTO IT, AS IN THIS ITALIAN-STYLE ROAST FLAVORED WITH PARSLEY, FENNEL, OREGANO, GARLIC, AND SPICY CRUSHED RED PEPPER.

- 2 tablespoons dried parsley, crushed
- 2 tablespoons fennel seeds, crushed
- 4 teaspoons dried oregano, crushed
- 1 teaspoon freshly ground black pepper
- ½ teaspoon crushed red pepper
- 4 cloves garlic, minced
- 1 4-pound bone-in pork shoulder roast
- 1 to 2 tablespoons olive oil
- 1¼ cups water
- 2 medium onions, peeled and cut into wedges
- 1 large fennel bulb, trimmed, cored, and cut into wedges
- 2 pounds Brussels sprouts

1. Preheat oven to 325°F. In a small bowl combine parsley, fennel seeds, oregano, black pepper, crushed red pepper, and garlic; set aside. Untie pork roast if necessary. Trim fat from meat. Rub the meat on all sides with the seasoning mixture. If desired, retie roast to hold it together.

2. In a Dutch oven heat oil over medium-high heat. Brown meat on all sides in the hot oil. Drain off fat. Pour the water into Dutch oven around roast. Roast, uncovered, for 1½ hours. Arrange onions and fennel around pork roast. Cover and roast for 30 minutes more.

3. Meanwhile, trim Brussels sprouts stems and remove any wilted outer leaves. Cut Brussels sprouts in half. Add Brussels sprouts to Dutch oven, arranging them over other vegetables. Cover and roast for 30 to 35 minutes more or until vegetables and meat are tender. Transfer meat to a serving platter and cover with foil. Let stand for 15 minutes before slicing. Toss vegetables with pan juices to coat. Using a slotted spoon, remove vegetables to the serving platter or a bowl; cover to keep warm.

4. Using a large spoon, skim fat from pan juices. Pour remaining pan juices through a sieve. Slice pork, removing the bone. Serve meat with vegetables and pan juices.

SLOW COOKER PORK MOLE

PREP: 20 minutes SLOW COOK: 8 to 10 hours (low) or 4 to 5 hours (high) MAKES: 8 servings

WITH CUMIN, CORIANDER, OREGANO, TOMATOES, ALMONDS, RAISINS, CHILE, AND CHOCOLATE, THIS RICH AND SPICY SAUCE HAS A LOT GOING ON—IN A VERY GOOD WAY. IT'S AN IDEAL MEAL TO START IN THE MORNING BEFORE YOU HEAD OUT FOR THE DAY. WHEN YOU COME HOME, DINNER IS NEARLY DONE— AND YOUR HOUSE SMELLS AMAZING.

- 1 3-pound boneless pork shoulder roast
- 1 cup coarsely chopped onion
- 3 cloves garlic, sliced
- 1½ cups Beef Bone Broth (see recipe), Chicken Bone Broth (see recipe), or no-salt-added beef or chicken broth
- 1 tablespoon ground cumin
- 1 tablespoon ground coriander
- 2 teaspoons dried oregano, crushed
- 1 15-ounce can diced no-salt-added tomatoes, drained
- 1 6-ounce can no-salt-added tomato paste
- ½ cup slivered almonds, toasted (see tip)
- ¼ cup unsulfured golden raisins or currants
- 2 ounces unsweetened chocolate (such as Scharffen Berger 99% cacao bar), coarsely chopped
- 1 dried whole ancho or chipotle chile pepper
- 2 4-inch cinnamon sticks
- ¼ cup snipped fresh cilantro
- 1 avocado, peeled, seeded, and thinly sliced
- 1 lime, cut into wedges
- ⅓ cup toasted unsalted green pumpkin seeds (optional) (see tip)

1. Trim fat from pork roast. If necessary, cut meat to fit a 5- to 6-quart slow cooker; set aside.

2. In the slow cooker combine onion and garlic. In a 2-cup glass measuring cup stir together Beef Bone Broth, cumin, coriander, and oregano; pour into cooker. Stir in diced tomatoes, tomato paste, almonds, raisins, chocolate, dried chile pepper, and cinnamon sticks. Place meat in cooker. Spoon some of the tomato mixture over the top. Cover and cook on low-heat setting for 8 to 10 hours or on high-heat setting for 4 to 5 hours or until pork is tender.

3. Transfer pork to a cutting board; cool slightly. Using two forks, pull meat apart into shreds. Cover meat with foil and set aside.

4. Remove and discard dried chile pepper and cinnamon sticks. Using a large spoon, skim fat from tomato mixture. Transfer the tomato mixture to a blender or food processor. Cover and blend or process until almost smooth. Return pulled pork and sauce into slow cooker. Keep warm on low-heat setting until serving time, up to 2 hours.

5. Just before serving, stir in cilantro. Serve mole in bowls and garnish with avocado slices, lime wedges, and, if desired, pumpkin seeds.

CARAWAY-SPICED PORK AND SQUASH STEW

PREP: 30 minutes COOK: 1 hour MAKES: 4 servings

PEPPERY MUSTARD GREENS AND BUTTERNUT SQUASH ADD VIBRANT COLOR AND A WHOLE HOST OF VITAMINS—AS WELL AS FIBER AND FOLIC ACID—TO THIS STEW SPICED WITH EASTERN EUROPEAN FLAVORS.

- 1 1¼- to 1½-pound pork shoulder roast
- 1 tablespoon paprika
- 1 tablespoon caraway seeds, finely crushed
- 2 teaspoons dry mustard
- ¼ teaspoon cayenne pepper
- 2 tablespoon refined coconut oil
- 8 ounces fresh button mushrooms, thinly sliced
- 2 stalks celery, cut crosswise into 1-inch slices
- 1 small red onion, cut into thin wedges
- 6 cloves garlic, minced
- 5 cups Chicken Bone Broth (see recipe) or no-salt-added chicken broth
- 2 cups cubed, peeled butternut squash
- 3 cups coarsely chopped, trimmed mustard greens or green cabbage
- 2 tablespoons snipped fresh sage
- ¼ cup fresh lemon juice

1. Trim fat from pork. Cut pork into 1½-inch cubes; place in a large bowl. In a small bowl combine paprika, caraway seeds, dry mustard, and cayenne pepper. Sprinkle over pork, tossing to coat evenly.

2. In a 4- to 5-quart Dutch oven heat coconut oil over medium heat. Add half of the meat; cook until browned, stirring

occasionally. Remove meat from the pan. Repeat with the remaining meat. Set meat aside.

3. Add mushrooms, celery, red onion, and garlic to Dutch oven. Cook for 5 minutes, stirring occasionally. Return meat to the Dutch oven. Carefully add Chicken Bone Broth. Bring to boiling; reduce heat. Cover and simmer for 45 minutes. Stir in squash. Cover and simmer for 10 to 15 minutes more or until pork and squash are tender. Stir in mustard greens and sage. Cook for 2 to 3 minutes or until greens are just tender. Stir in lemon juice.

FRUIT-STUFFED TOP LOIN ROAST WITH BRANDY SAUCE

PREP: 30 minutes COOK: 10 minutes ROAST: 1 hour 15 minutes STAND: 15 minutes MAKES: 8 to 10 servings

THIS ELEGANT ROAST IS PERFECT FOR A SPECIAL OCCASION OR FAMILY GATHERING—PARTICULARLY IN THE FALL. ITS FLAVORS—APPLES, NUTMEG, DRIED FRUIT, AND PECANS—CAPTURE THE ESSENCE OF THAT SEASON. SERVE IT WITH MASHED SWEET POTATOES AND BLUEBERRY AND ROASTED BEET KALE SALAD (SEE RECIPE).

ROAST
- 1 tablespoon olive oil
- 2 cups chopped, peeled Granny Smith apples (about 2 medium)
- 1 shallot, finely chopped
- 1 tablespoon snipped fresh thyme
- ¾ teaspoon freshly ground black pepper
- ⅛ teaspoon ground nutmeg
- ½ cup snipped unsulfured dried apricots
- ¼ cup chopped pecans, toasted (see tip)
- 1 cup Chicken Bone Broth (see recipe) or no-salt-added chicken broth
- 1 3-pound boneless pork top loin roast (single loin)

BRANDY SAUCE
- 2 tablespoons apple cider
- 2 tablespoons brandy
- 1 teaspoon Dijon-Style Mustard (see recipe)
- Freshly ground black pepper

1. For the stuffing, in a large skillet heat olive oil over medium heat. Add apples, shallot, thyme, ¼ teaspoon of the pepper, and nutmeg; cook for 2 to 4 minutes or until

apples and shallot are tender and light golden, stirring occasionally. Stir in apricots, pecans, and 1 tablespoon of the broth. Cook, uncovered, for 1 minute to soften apricots. Remove from heat and set aside.

2. Preheat oven to 325°F. Butterfly the pork roast by making a lengthwise cut down the center of the roast, cutting to within ½ inch of the other side. Spread the roast open. Place the knife in the V cut, facing it horizontally toward one side of the V, and cut to within ½ inch of the side. Repeat on the other side of the V. Spread the roast open and cover with plastic wrap. Working from the center to the edges, pound the roast with a meat mallet until it is about ¾ inch thick. Remove and discard plastic wrap. Spread the stuffing over the top of the roast. Starting from a short side, roll the roast into a spiral. Tie with 100%-cotton kitchen string in several places to hold the roast together. Sprinkle roast with the remaining ½ teaspoon pepper.

3. Place roast on a rack in a shallow roasting pan. Insert an oven-going thermometer into the center of the roast (not in the stuffing). Roast, uncovered, for 1 hour 15 minutes to 1 hour 30 minutes or until thermometer registers 145°F. Remove roast and cover loosely with foil; let stand for 15 minutes before slicing.

4. Meanwhile, for Brandy Sauce, stir the remaining broth and apple cider into drippings in pan, whisking to scrape up browned bits. Strain drippings into a medium saucepan. Bring to boiling; cook about 4 minutes or until sauce is reduced by one-third. Stir in brandy and Dijon-Style

Mustard. Season to taste with additional pepper. Serve sauce with the pork roast.

PORCHETTA-STYLE PORK ROAST

PREP: 15 minutes MARINATE: overnight STAND: 40 minutes ROAST: 1 hour MAKES: 6 servings

TRADITIONAL ITALIAN PORCHETTA (SOMETIMES SPELLED PORKETTA IN AMERICAN ENGLISH) IS A BONELESS SUCKLING PIG STUFFED WITH GARLIC, FENNEL, PEPPER, AND HERBS SUCH AS SAGE OR ROSEMARY, THEN PUT ON A SPIT AND ROASTED OVER WOOD. IT'S ALSO USUALLY HEAVILY SALTED. THIS PALEO VERSION IS SIMPLIFIED AND VERY TASTY. SUBSTITUTE FRESH ROSEMARY FOR THE SAGE, IF YOU LIKE, OR USE A BLEND OF THE TWO HERBS.

- 1 2- to 3-pound boneless pork loin roast
- 2 tablespoons fennel seeds
- 1 teaspoon black peppercorns
- ½ teaspoon crushed red pepper
- 6 cloves garlic, minced
- 1 tablespoon finely shredded orange peel
- 1 tablespoon snipped fresh sage
- 3 tablespoon olive oil
- ½ cup dry white wine
- ½ cup Chicken Bone Broth (see recipe) or no-salt-added chicken broth

1. Remove pork roast from refrigerator; let stand at room temperature for 30 minutes. Meanwhile, in a small skillet toast fennel seeds over medium heat, stirring frequently, about 3 minutes or until dark in color and fragrant; cool. Transfer to a spice mill or clean coffee grinder. Add peppercorns and crushed red pepper. Grind to medium-fine consistency. (Do not grind to a powder.)

2. Preheat oven to 325°F. In a small bowl combine ground spices, garlic, orange peel, sage, and olive oil to make a paste. Place pork roast on a rack in a small roasting pan. Rub mixture all over pork. (If desired, place seasoned pork in a 9×13×2-inch glass baking dish. Cover with with plastic wrap and refrigerate overnight to marinate. Transfer meat to a roasting pan before cooking and let stand at room temperature for 30 minutes before cooking.)

3. Roast pork for 1 to 1½ hours or until an instant-read thermometer inserted into center of roast registers 145°F. Transfer roast to a cutting board and cover loosely with foil. Let stand for 10 to 15 minutes before slicing.

4. Meanwhile, pour pan juices into a glass measuring cup. Skim fat from top; set aside. Place roasting pan on stovetop burner. Pour wine and Chicken Bone Broth into pan. Bring to boiling over medium-high heat, stirring to scrape up any browned bits. Boil about 4 minutes or until mixture is slightly reduced. Whisk in reserved pan juices; strain. Slice pork and serve with sauce.

TOMATILLO-BRAISED PORK LOIN

PREP: 40 minutes BROIL: 10 minutes COOK: 20 minutes ROAST: 40 minutes STAND: 10 minutes MAKES: 6 to 8 servings

TOMATILLOS HAVE A STICKY, SAPPY COATING UNDER THEIR PAPER SKINS. AFTER YOU REMOVE THE SKINS, GIVE THEM A QUICK RINSE UNDER RUNNING WATER AND THEY ARE READY TO USE.

- 1 pound tomatillos, husked, stemmed, and rinsed
- 4 serrano chiles, stemmed, seeded, and halved (see tip)
- 2 jalapeños, stemmed, seeded, and halved (see tip)
- 1 large yellow sweet pepper, stemmed, seeded, and halved
- 1 large orange sweet pepper, stemmed, seeded, and halved
- 2 tablespoons olive oil
- 1 2- to 2½-pound boneless pork loin roast
- 1 large yellow onion, peeled, halved, and thinly sliced
- 4 cloves garlic, minced
- ¾ cup water
- ¼ cup fresh lime juice
- ¼ cup snipped fresh cilantro

1. Preheat broiler to high. Line a baking sheet with foil. Arrange tomatillos, serrano chiles, jalapeños, and sweet peppers on prepared baking sheet. Broil vegetables 4 inches from heat until well charred, turning tomatillos occasionally and removing vegetables as they become charred, about 10 to 15 minutes. Place serranos, jalapeños, and tomatillos in a bowl. Place sweet peppers on a plate. Set vegetables aside to cool.

2. In a large skillet heat oil over medium-high heat until it shimmers. Pat pork roast dry with clean paper towels and add to skillet. Cook until well browned on all sides,

turning roast to brown evenly. Transfer roast to a platter. Reduce heat to medium. Add onion to skillet; cook and stir for 5 to 6 minutes or until golden. Add garlic; cook for 1 minute more. Remove skillet from heat.

3. Preheat oven to 350°F. For tomatillo sauce, in a food processor or blender combine tomatillos, serranos, and jalapeños. Cover and blend or process until smooth; add to onion in skillet. Return skillet to heat. Bring to boiling; cook for 4 to 5 minutes or until mixture is dark and thick. Stir in the water, lime juice, and cilantro.

4. Spread tomatillo sauce in a shallow roasting pan or 3-quart rectangular baking dish. Place pork roast in the sauce. Cover tightly with foil. Roast for 40 to 45 minutes or until an instant-read thermometer inserted into the center of the roast reads 140°F.

5. Cut sweet peppers into strips. Stir into the tomatillo sauce in pan. Tent loosely with foil; let stand for 10 minutes. Slice meat; stir sauce. Serve sliced pork topped generously with tomatillo sauce.

APRICOT-STUFFED PORK TENDERLOIN

PREP: 20 minutes ROAST: 45 minutes STAND: 5 minutes MAKES: 2 to 3 servings

- 2 medium fresh apricots, coarsely chopped
- 2 tablespoons unsulfured raisins
- 2 tablespoons chopped walnuts
- 2 teaspoons grated fresh ginger
- ¼ teaspoon ground cardamom
- 1 12-ounce pork tenderloin
- 1 tablespoon olive oil
- 1 tablespoon Dijon-Style Mustard (see recipe)
- ¼ teaspoon black pepper

1. Preheat oven to 375°F. Line a baking sheet with foil; place a roasting rack on the baking sheet.

2. In a small bowl stir together the apricots, raisins, walnuts, ginger, and cardamom.

3. Make a lengthwise cut down the center of the pork, cutting to within ½ inch of the other side. Butterfly it open. Place the pork between two layers of plastic wrap. Using the flat side of a meat mallet, lightly pound meat until about ⅓ inch thick. Fold in the tail end to make an even rectangle. Lightly pound meat to make even thickness.

4. Spread the apricot mixture over the pork. Beginning at the narrow end, roll up the pork. Tie with 100%-cotton kitchen string, first in the center, then at 1-inch intervals. Place roast on the rack.

5. Stir together the olive oil and Dijon-Style Mustard; brush over the roast. Sprinkle roast with pepper. Roast for 45 to

55 minutes or until an instant-read thermometer inserted into center of roast registers 140°F. Let stand for 5 to 10 minutes before slicing.

HERB-CRUSTED PORK TENDERLOIN WITH CRISPY GARLIC OIL

PREP: 15 minutes ROAST: 30 minutes COOK: 8 minutes STAND: 5 minutes MAKES: 6 servings

⅓ cup Dijon-Style Mustard (see recipe)
¼ cup snipped fresh parsley
2 tablespoons snipped fresh thyme
1 tablespoon snipped fresh rosemary
½ teaspoon black pepper
2 12-ounce pork tenderloins
½ cup olive oil
¼ cup minced fresh garlic
¼ to 1 teaspoon crushed red pepper

1. Preheat oven to 450°F. Line a baking sheet with foil; place a roasting rack on the baking sheet.

2. In a small bowl stir together the mustard, parsley, thyme, rosemary, and black pepper to make a paste. Spread the mustard-herb mixture over the top and sides of the pork. Transfer pork to the roasting rack. Place roast in the oven; decrease temperature to 375°F. Roast for 30 to 35 minutes or until an instant-read thermometer inserted into center of roast registers 140°F. Let stand for 5 to 10 minutes before slicing.

3. Meanwhile, for garlic oil, in a small saucepan combine the olive oil and garlic. Cook over medium-low heat for 8 to 10 minutes or until garlic is golden and begins to crisp (do not let garlic burn). Remove from heat; stir in crushed red pepper. Slice pork; spoon garlic oil over the slices before serving.

INDIAN-SPICED PORK WITH COCONUT PAN SAUCE

START TO FINISH: 20 minutes MAKES: 2 servings

- 3 teaspoons curry powder
- 2 teaspoons salt-free garam masala
- 1 teaspoon ground cumin
- 1 teaspoon ground coriander
- 1 12-ounce pork tenderloin
- 1 tablespoon olive oil
- ½ cup natural coconut milk (such as Nature's Way brand)
- ¼ cup snipped fresh cilantro
- 2 tablespoons snipped fresh mint

1. In a small bowl stir together 2 teaspoons of the curry powder, garam masala, cumin, and coriander. Slice pork into ½-inch-thick slices; sprinkle with spices. .

2. In a large skillet heat olive oil over medium heat. Add pork slices to skillet; cook for 7 minutes, turning once. Remove pork from skillet; cover to keep warm. For sauce, add coconut milk and the remaining 1 teaspoon curry powder to the skillet, stirring to scrape up any bits. Simmer for 2 to 3 minutes. Stir in cilantro and mint. Add pork; cook until heated through, spooning sauce over the pork.

PORK SCALOPPINI WITH SPICED APPLES AND CHESTNUTS

PREP: 20 minutes COOK: 15 minutes MAKES: 4 servings

2 12-ounce pork tenderloins
1 tablespoon onion powder
1 tablespoon garlic powder
½ teaspoon black pepper
2 to 4 tablespoons olive oil
2 Fuji or Pink Lady apples, peeled, cored, and coarsely chopped
¼ cup finely chopped shallots
¾ teaspoon ground cinnamon
⅛ teaspoon ground cloves
⅛ teaspoon ground nutmeg
½ cup Chicken Bone Broth (see recipe) or no-salt added chicken broth
2 tablespoons fresh lemon juice
½ cup peeled roasted chestnuts, chopped,* or chopped pecans
1 tablespoon snipped fresh sage

1. Cut the tenderloins into ½-inch- thick slices on a bias. Place pork slices between two sheets of plastic wrap. Using the flat side of a meat mallet, pound until thin. Sprinkle slices with onion powder, garlic powder, and black pepper.

2. In a large skillet heat 2 tablespoons olive oil over medium heat. Cook pork, in batches, for 3 to 4 minutes, turning once and adding oil if necessary. Transfer pork to a plate; cover and keep warm.

3. Increase heat to medium-high. Add the apples, shallots, cinnamon, cloves, and nutmeg. Cook and stir for 3 minutes. Stir in Chicken Bone Broth and lemon juice.

Cover and cook for 5 minutes. Remove from heat; stir in the chestnuts and sage. Serve apple mixture over pork.

*Note: To roast chestnuts, preheat oven to 400°F. Cut an X in one side of the chestnut shell. This will let the shell loosen as it cooks. Place chestnuts on a baking pan and roast for 30 minutes or until the shell pulls apart from the nut and the nuts are tender. Wrap the roasted chestnuts in a clean kitchen towel. Peel shells and skin from the yellow-white nut.

PORK FAJITA STIR-FRY

PREP: 20 minutes COOK: 22 minutes MAKES: 4 servings

1 pound pork tenderloin, cut into 2-inch strips
3 tablespoons salt-free fajita seasoning or Mexican Seasoning (see recipe)
2 tablespoons olive oil
1 small onion, thinly sliced
½ of a red sweet pepper, seeded and thinly sliced
½ of an orange sweet pepper, seeded and thinly sliced
1 jalapeño, stemmed and thinly sliced (see tip) (optional)
½ teaspoon cumin seeds
1 cup thinly sliced fresh mushrooms
3 tablespoons fresh lime juice
½ cup snipped fresh cilantro
1 avocado, seeded, peeled, and diced
Desired salsa (see recipes)

1. Sprinkle the pork with 2 tablespoons fajita seasoning. In an extra-large skillet heat 1 tablespoon of the oil over medium-high heat. Add half the pork; cook and stir about 5 minutes or until no longer pink. Transfer meat to a bowl and cover to keep warm. Repeat with remaining oil and pork.

2. Turn heat to medium. Add the remaining 1 tablespoon fajita seasoning, onion, sweet peppers, jalapeño, and cumin. Cook and stir about 10 minutes or until vegetables are tender. Return all the meat and accumulated juices to skillet. Stir in mushrooms and lime juice. Cook until heated through. Remove skillet from heat; stir in the cilantro. Serve with avocado and desired salsa.

PORK TENDERLOIN WITH PORT AND PRUNES

PREP: 10 minutes ROAST: 12 minutes STAND: 5 minutes MAKES: 4 servings

PORT IS A FORTIFIED WINE, WHICH MEANS IT HAS A SPIRIT SIMILAR TO BRANDY ADDED TO IT TO STOP THE FERMENTATION PROCESS. THIS MEANS THERE IS MORE RESIDUAL SUGAR IN IT THAN RED TABLE WINE AND CONSEQUENTLY IT HAS A SWEETER TASTE. IT ISN'T SOMETHING YOU WANT TO DRINK EVERY DAY, BUT A LITTLE BIT USED IN COOKING ONCE IN A WHILE IS FINE.

- 2 12-ounce pork tenderloins
- 2½ teaspoons ground coriander
- ¼ teaspoon black pepper
- 2 tablespoons olive oil
- 1 shallot, sliced
- ½ cup port wine
- ½ cup Chicken Bone Broth (see recipe) or no-salt-added chicken broth
- 20 pitted unsulfured dried plums (prunes)
- ½ teaspoon crushed red pepper
- 2 teaspoons snipped fresh tarragon

1. Preheat oven to 400°F. Sprinkle pork with 2 teaspoons of the coriander and the black pepper.

2. In a large ovenproof skillet heat olive oil over medium-high heat. Add tenderloins to skillet. Cook until browned on all sides, turning to brown evenly, about 8 minutes. Place skillet in oven. Roast, uncovered, about 12 minutes or until an instant-read thermometer inserted into center of roasts registers 140°F. Transfer tenderloins to a cutting

board. Cover loosely with aluminum foil and let stand for 5 minutes.

3. Meanwhile, for sauce, drain fat from skillet, reserving 1 tablespoon. Cook shallot in the reserved drippings in skillet over medium heat about 3 minutes or until browned and tender. Add port to skillet. Bring to boiling, stirring to scrape up any browned bits. Add Chicken Bone Broth, dried plums, crushed red pepper, and the remaining ½ teaspoon coriander. Cook over medium-high heat to reduce slightly, about 1 to 2 minutes. Stir in tarragon.

4. Slice pork and serve with prunes and sauce.

MOO SHU-STYLE PORK IN LETTUCE CUPS WITH QUICK PICKLED VEGETABLES

START TO FINISH: 45 minutes MAKES: 4 servings

IF YOU'VE HAD A TRADITIONAL MOO SHU DISH IN A CHINESE RESTAURANT, YOU KNOW IT IS A SAVORY MEAT AND VEGETABLE FILLING EATEN IN THIN PANCAKES WITH A SWEET PLUM OR HOISIN SAUCE. THIS LIGHTER AND FRESHER PALEO VERSION FEATURES PORK, CHINESE CABBAGE, AND SHIITAKE MUSHROOMS STIR-FRIED IN GINGER AND GARLIC AND ENJOYED IN LETTUCE WRAPS WITH CRUNCHY PICKLED VEGETABLES.

PICKLED VEGETABLES
- 1 cup julienne-cut carrots
- 1 cup julienne-cut daikon radish
- ¼ cup slivered red onion
- 1 cup unsweetened apple juice
- ½ cup cider vinegar

PORK
- 2 tablespoons olive oil or refined coconut oil
- 3 eggs, lightly beaten
- 8 ounces pork loin, cut into 2×½-inch strips
- 2 teaspoons minced fresh ginger
- 4 cloves garlic, minced
- 2 cups thinly sliced napa cabbage
- 1 cup thinly sliced shiitake mushrooms
- ¼ cup thinly sliced scallions
- 8 Boston lettuce leaves

1. For quick pickled vegetables, in a large bowl toss together the carrots, daikon, and onion. For brine, in a saucepan heat the apple juice and vinegar just until steam rises. Pour the brine over the vegetables in bowl; cover and chill until ready to serve.

2. In a large skillet heat 1 tablespoon of the oil over medium-high heat. Using a whisk, lightly beat eggs. Add eggs to skillet; cook, without stirring, until set on the bottom, about 3 minutes. Using a flexible spatula, carefully turn the egg over and cook on the other side. Slide the egg out of the pan onto a platter.

3. Return the skillet to heat; add the remaining 1 tablespoon oil. Add the pork strips, ginger, and garlic. Cook and stir over medium-high heat about 4 minutes or until pork is no longer pink. Add the cabbage and mushrooms; cook and stir about 4 minutes or until cabbage wilts, mushrooms soften, and pork is cooked through. Remove skillet from heat. Cut the cooked egg into strips. Gently stir egg strips and scallions into pork mixture. Serve in lettuce leaves and top with pickled vegetables.

PORK CHOPS WITH MACADAMIAS, SAGE, FIGS, AND MASHED SWEET POTATOES

PREP: 15 minutes COOK: 25 minutes MAKES: 4 servings

PAIRED WITH MASHED SWEET POTATOES, THESE JUICY SAGE-TOPPED CHOPS MAKE A PERFECT FALL MEAL—AND ONE THAT'S QUICK TO FIX, MAKING IT A PERFECT FOR A BUSY WEEKNIGHT.

- 4 boneless pork loin chops, cut 1¼ inches thick
- 3 tablespoons snipped fresh sage
- ¼ teaspoon black pepper
- 3 tablespoons macadamia nut oil
- 2 pounds sweet potatoes, peeled and cut into 1-inch pieces
- ¾ cup chopped macadamia nuts
- ½ cup chopped dried figs
- ⅓ cup Beef Bone Broth (see recipe) or no-salt-added beef broth
- 1 tablespoon fresh lemon juice

1. Sprinkle both sides of pork chops with 2 tablespoons of the sage and the pepper; rub in with your fingers. In a large skillet heat 2 tablespoons of the oil over medium heat. Add chops to skillet; cook for 15 to 20 minutes or until done (145°F), turning once halfway through cooking. Transfer chops to a plate; cover to keep warm.

2. Meanwhile, in a large saucepan combine sweet potatoes and enough water to cover. Bring to boiling; reduce heat. Cover and simmer for 10 to 15 minutes or until potatoes are tender. Drain potatoes. Add the remaining tablespoon macadamia oil to potatoes and mash until creamy; keep warm.

3. For sauce, add macadamia nuts to skillet; cook over medium heat just until toasted. Add dried figs and the remaining 1 tablespoon sage; cook for 30 seconds. Add Beef Bone Broth and lemon juice to skillet, stirring to scrape up any browned bits. Spoon sauce over pork chops and serve with mashed sweet potatoes.

SKILLET-ROASTED ROSEMARY-LAVENDER PORK CHOPS WITH GRAPES AND TOASTED WALNUTS

PREP: 10 minutes COOK: 6 minutes ROAST: 25 minutes MAKES: 4 servings

ROASTING THE GRAPES ALONG WITH THE PORK CHOPS INTENSIFIES THEIR FLAVOR AND SWEETNESS. ALONG WITH THE CRUNCHY TOASTED WALNUTS AND A SPRINKLING OF FRESH ROSEMARY, THEY MAKE A WONDERFUL TOPPING FOR THESE HEARTY CHOPS.

2 tablespoons snipped fresh rosemary

1 tablespoon snipped fresh lavender

½ teaspoon garlic powder

½ teaspoon black pepper

4 pork loin chops, cut 1¼ inches thick (about 3 pounds)

1 tablespoon olive oil

1 large shallot, thinly sliced

1½ cups red and/or green seedless grapes

½ cup dry white wine

¾ cup coarsely chopped walnuts

Snipped fresh rosemary

1. Preheat oven to 375°F. In a small bowl combine 2 tablespoons rosemary, lavender, garlic powder, and pepper. Rub herb mixture evenly into pork chops. In an extra-large ovenproof skillet heat olive oil over medium heat. Add chops to skillet; cook for 6 to 8 minutes or until browned on both sides. Transfer chops to a plate; cover with foil.

2. Add the shallot to the skillet. Cook and stir over medium heat for 1 minute. Add grapes and wine. Cook about 2 minutes more, stirring to scrape up any browned bits. Return pork chops to skillet. Place the skillet in the oven; roast for 25 to 30 minutes or until chops are done (145°F).

3. Meanwhile, spread the walnuts in a shallow baking pan. Add to oven with chops. Roast about 8 minutes or until toasted, stirring once to toast evenly.

4. To serve, top pork chops with grapes and toasted walnuts. Sprinkle with additional fresh rosemary.

PORK CHOPS ALLA FIORENTINA WITH GRILLED BROCCOLI RABE

PREP: 20 minutes GRILL: 20 minutes MARINATE: 3 minutes MAKES: 4 servings PHOTO

"ALLA FIORENTINA" ESSENTIALLY MEANS "IN THE STYLE OF FLORENCE." THIS RECIPE IS STYLED AFTER *BISTECCA ALLA FIORENTINA*, A TUSCAN T-BONE GRILLED OVER A WOOD FIRE WITH THE SIMPLEST FLAVORINGS—USUALLY JUST OLIVE OIL, SALT, BLACK PEPPER, AND A SQUEEZE OF FRESH LEMON TO FINISH.

- 1 pound broccoli rabe
- 1 tablespoon olive oil
- 4 6- to 8-ounce bone-in pork loin chops, cut 1½ to 2 inches thick
- Coarsely ground black pepper
- 1 lemon
- 4 cloves garlic, thinly sliced
- 2 tablespoons snipped fresh rosemary
- 6 fresh sage leaves, chopped
- 1 teaspoon crushed red pepper flakes (or to taste)
- ½ cup olive oil

1. In a large saucepan blanch the broccoli rabe in boiling water for 1 minute. Immediately transfer to a bowl of ice water. When cool, drain the broccoli rabe on a paper towel-lined baking sheet, blotting as dry as possible with additional paper towels. Remove paper towels from baking sheet. Drizzle the broccoli rabe with 1 tablespoon olive oil, tossing to coat; set aside until ready to grill.

2. Sprinkle both sides of the pork chops with coarsely ground pepper; set aside. Using a vegetable peeler, remove strips

of peel from lemon (save lemon for another use). Scatter lemon peel strips, sliced garlic, rosemary, sage, and crushed red pepper on a large serving platter; set aside.

3. For a charcoal grill, move most hot coals to one side of the grill, leaving some coals under the other side of the grill. Sear the chops directly over the hot coals for 2 to 3 minutes or until a brown crust forms. Turn the chops over and sear on the second side for 2 minutes more. Move the chops to the other side of the grill. Cover and grill for 10 to 15 minutes or until done (145°F). (For a gas grill, preheat grill; reduce heat on one side of grill to medium. Sear chops as directed above over high heat. Move to medium heat side of grill; continue as directed above.)

4. Transfer the chops to the platter. Drizzle chops with the ½ cup olive oil, turning to coat both sides. Let the chops marinate for 3 to 5 minutes before serving, turning once or twice to infuse the meat with the flavors of the lemon peel, garlic, and herbs.

5. While the chops rest, grill the broccoli rabe to char lightly and warm through. Arrange broccoli rabe on the platter with the pork chops; spoon some of the marinade over each chop and broccoli rabe before serving.

ESCAROLE-STUFFED PORK CHOPS

PREP: 20 minutes COOK: 9 minutes MAKES: 4 servings

ESCAROLE CAN BE EATEN AS A SALAD GREEN OR LIGHTLY SAUTÉED WITH GARLIC IN OLIVE OIL FOR A QUICK SIDE DISH. HERE, COMBINED WITH OLIVE OIL, GARLIC, BLACK PEPPER, CRUSHED RED PEPPER, AND LEMON, IT MAKES A BEAUTIFUL BRIGHT-GREEN FILLING FOR JUICY PAN-SEARED PORK CHOPS.

4 6- to 8-ounce bone-in pork chops, cut ¾ inch thick
½ of a medium head escarole, finely chopped
4 tablespoons olive oil
1 tablespoon fresh lemon juice
¼ teaspoon black pepper
¼ teaspoon crushed red pepper
2 large cloves garlic, minced
Olive oil
1 tablespoon snipped fresh sage
¼ teaspoon black pepper
⅓ cup dry white wine

1. Using a paring knife, cut a deep pocket, about 2 inches wide, into the curved side of each pork chop; set aside.

2. In a large bowl combine escarole, 2 tablespoons of the olive oil, lemon juice, ¼ teaspoon black pepper, crushed red pepper, and garlic. Stuff each chop with one-fourth of the mixture. Brush chops with olive oil. Sprinkle with sage and ¼ teaspoon ground black pepper.

3. In an extra-large skillet heat remaining 2 tablespoons olive oil over medium-high heat. Sear pork for 4 minutes on each side until golden brown. Transfer chops to a plate.

Add wine to skillet, scraping up any browned bits. Reduce pan juices for 1 minute.

4. Drizzle chops with pan juices before serving.

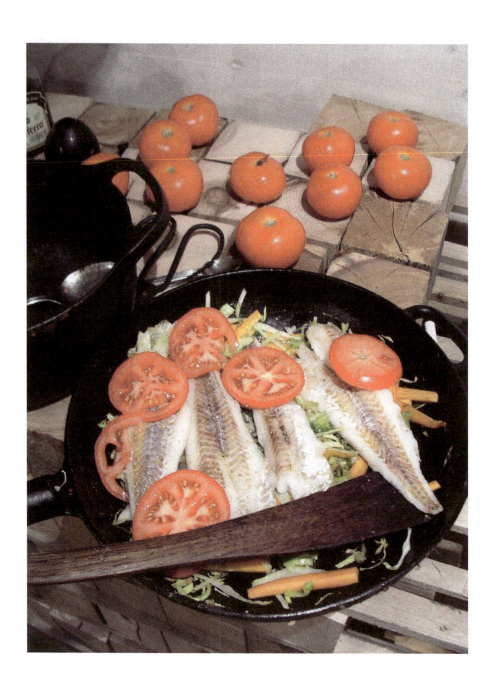

PORK CHOPS WITH A DIJON-PECAN CRUST

PREP: 15 minutes COOK: 6 minutes BAKE: 3 minutes MAKES: 4 servings PHOTO

THESE MUSTARD-AND-NUT-CRUSTED CHOPS COULDN'T BE SIMPLER TO MAKE—AND THE TASTE PAY-OFF FAR EXCEEDS THE EFFORT. TRY THEM WITH CINNAMON-ROASTED BUTTERNUT SQUASH (SEE RECIPE), NEO-CLASSIC WALDORF SALAD (SEE RECIPE), OR BRUSSELS SPROUTS AND APPLE SALAD (SEE RECIPE).

⅓ cup finely chopped pecans, toasted (see tip)
1 tablespoon snipped fresh sage
3 tablespoons olive oil
4 bone-in center-cut pork chops, about 1 inch thick (about 2 pounds total)
½ teaspoon black pepper
2 tablespoons olive oil
3 tablespoons Dijon-Style Mustard (see recipe)

1. Preheat oven to 400°F. In a small bowl combine pecans, sage, and 1 tablespoon of the olive oil.

2. Sprinkle pork chops with pepper. In a large ovenproof skillet heat the remaining 2 tablespoons olive oil over high heat. Add chops; cook about 6 minutes or until browned on both sides, turning once. Remove skillet from heat. Spread Dijon-Style Mustard on tops of chops; sprinkle with pecan mixture, lightly pressing into mustard.

3. Place skillet in oven. Bake for 3 to 4 minutes or until chops are done (145°F).

WALNUT-CRUSTED PORK WITH BLACKBERRY SPINACH SALAD

PREP: 30 minutes COOK: 4 minutes MAKES: 4 servings

PORK HAS A NATURALLY SWEET TASTE THAT PAIRS WELL WITH FRUIT. ALTHOUGH THE USUAL SUSPECTS ARE FALL FRUITS SUCH AS APPLES AND PEARS—OR STONE FRUITS SUCH AS PEACHES, PLUMS, AND APRICOTS—PORK IS ALSO DELICIOUS WITH BLACKBERRIES, WHICH HAVE A SWEET-TART, WINELIKE FLAVOR.

- 1⅔ cups blackberries
- 1 tablespoon plus 1½ teaspoons water
- 3 tablespoons walnut oil
- 1 tablespoon plus 1½ teaspoons white wine vinegar
- 2 eggs
- ¾ cup almond meal
- ⅓ cup finely chopped walnuts
- 1 tablespoon plus 1½ teaspoons Mediterranean Seasoning (see recipe)
- 4 pork cutlets or boneless pork loin chops (1 to 1½ pounds total)
- 6 cups fresh baby spinach leaves
- ½ cup torn fresh basil leaves
- ½ cup slivered red onion
- ½ cup chopped walnuts, toasted (see tip)
- ¼ cup refined coconut oil

1. For blackberry vinaigrette, in a small saucepan combine 1 cup of the blackberries and the water. Bring to boiling; reduce heat. Simmer, covered, for 4 to 5 minutes or just until berries are softened and color turns to a bright maroon, stirring occasionally. Remove from the heat; cool slightly. Pour undrained blackberries into a blender or

food processor; cover and blend or process until smooth. Using the back of a spoon, press pureed berries through a fine-mesh sieve; discard seeds and solids. In a medium bowl whisk together strained berries, walnut oil, and vinegar; set aside.

2. Line a large baking sheet with parchment paper; set aside. In a shallow dish lightly beat eggs well with a fork. In another shallow dish combine almond meal, the ⅓ cup finely chopped walnuts, and Mediterranean Seasoning. Dip pork cutlets, one at a time, in eggs and then in walnut mixture, turning to coat evenly. Place coated pork cutlets on a prepared baking sheet; set aside.

3. In a large bowl combine spinach and basil. Divide greens among four serving plates, arranging them along one side of the plates. Top with remaining ⅔ cup berries, the red onion, and the ½ cup toasted walnuts. Drizzle with blackberry vinaigrette.

4. In an extra-large skillet heat coconut oil over medium-high heat. Add pork cutlets to skillet; cook about 4 minutes or until done (145°F), turning once. Add pork cutlets to plates with salad.

PORK SCHNITZEL WITH SWEET-AND-SOUR RED CABBAGE

PREP: 20 minutes COOK: 45 minutes MAKES: 4 servings

IN THE "PALEO PRINCIPLES" SECTION OF THIS BOOK, ALMOND FLOUR (ALSO CALLED ALMOND MEAL) IS LISTED AS A NON-PALEO INGREDIENT—NOT BECAUSE ALMOND FLOUR IS INHERENTLY BAD, BUT BECAUSE IT IS FREQUENTLY USED TO CREATE ANALOGS OF WHEAT-FLOUR BROWNIES, CAKES, COOKIES, ETC., THAT SHOULD NOT BE A REGULAR PART OF A REAL PALEO DIET®. USED IN MODERATION AS COATING FOR A THIN SCALLOP OF PAN-FRIED PORK OR POULTRY, AS IT IS HERE, IS NOT A PROBLEM.

CABBAGE

- 2 tablespoons olive oil
- 1 cup chopped red onion
- 6 cups thinly sliced red cabbage (about ½ of a head)
- 2 Granny Smith apples, peeled, cored, and diced
- ¾ cup fresh orange juice
- 3 tablespoons cider vinegar
- ½ teaspoon caraway seeds
- ½ teaspoon celery seeds
- ½ teaspoon black pepper

PORK

- 4 boneless pork loin chops, cut ½ inch thick
- 2 cups almond flour
- 1 tablespoon dried lemon peel
- 2 teaspoons black pepper
- ¾ teaspoon ground allspice
- 1 large egg

¼ cup almond milk
3 tablespoons olive oil
Lemon wedges

1. For sweet-and-sour cabbage, in a 6-quart Dutch oven heat olive oil over medium-low heat. Add onion; cook for 6 to 8 minutes or until tender and lightly browned. Add cabbage; cook and stir for 6 to 8 minutes or until cabbage is crisp-tender. Add apples, orange juice, vinegar, caraway seeds, celery seeds, and ½ teaspoon pepper. Bring to boiling; reduce heat to low. Cover and cook for 30 minutes, stirring occasionally. Uncover and cook until liquid is reduced slightly.

2. Meanwhile, for pork, place chops between two sheets of plastic wrap or waxed paper. Using the flat side of a meat mallet or rolling pin, pound to about ¼ inch thickness; set aside.

3. In a shallow dish combine almond flour, dried lemon peel, 2 teaspoons pepper, and allspice. In another shallow dish whisk together the egg and almond milk. Lightly coat the pork cutlets in the seasoned flour, shaking off excess. Dip in the egg mixture, then again into the seasoned flour, shaking off excess. Repeat with remaining cutlets.

4. In a large skillet heat olive oil over medium-high heat. Add 2 cutlets to the pan. Cook for 6 to 8 minutes or until cutlets are golden brown and cooked through, turning once. Transfer cutlets to a warm platter. Repeat with remaining 2 cutlets.

5. Serve cutlets with cabbage and lemon wedges.

Lightning Source UK Ltd.
Milton Keynes UK
UKHW020750220421
382423UK00001B/60